31 DAYS OF GOD'S WORD FOR *HEALTH*, *WHOLENESS*, AND *PEACE*

HEALING NUGGETS

31-DAY DEVOTIONAL

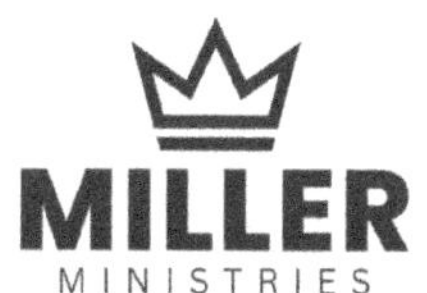

Healing Nuggets: 31 Days of God's Word for Health, Wholeness, and Peace
ISBN: 978-0-9846918-7-6

Published by:
Miller Ministries
4000 Westbrook Drive
Aurora, IL 60504 USA
(630) 851-4000
www.millerministries.org

Editorial Consultant: Anne Schreiber, Aurora, IL

Cover Design: Timothy Miller

Cover Photo: Seth Wheeler © Miller Ministries

Dedication

I lovingly dedicate this book to the congregation of Abundant Life Family Church. When I said "yes" to the plan of God to reach out on YouTube with the message of faith and healing, it became an entire church project. Thank you for joyfully taking this journey of faith with me into this new chapter of our ministry. I will always be grateful for the supply of prayer, faith, and encouragement that you bring!

Contents

Preface

Having worked as a registered nurse for many years, I have seen the good, the bad, and the ugly when it comes to sickness and disease. In over forty years of ministry, I have ministered to countless people who have suffered from all kinds of disease, pain, and mental torment. I will never be convinced that these were a blessing from God!

People long for health and healing more than almost anything else. Throughout the ages, mankind has been on a quest to find the fountain of youth and healing remedies when all along the answers have lied within the pages of our Bibles.

As you read these devotionals, you will get *daily nuggets* of scripture and teachings on healing that clearly show the will of God concerning sickness and disease. You will also notice a lot of repetition, because this is how faith comes. You will discover where sickness comes from, how to receive healing, and how to keep disease from coming back into your life.

My prayer is that you will begin to see how faithful God is to perform His Word in your life, and that *all* things are possible to you if you will only believe.

Christine Miller

Day 1

Where Does Sickness Come From?

Many have wondered where sickness comes from and why people are sick. These are very important questions that need clear scriptural answers. You see, in order to receive healing from God, the first thing that must be established is the origin of sickness and disease.

Jesus said, "The thief does not come except to steal, and to kill, and to destroy. I have come that they may have life, and that they may have it more abundantly" (John 10:10). This scripture reveals that anything that steals, kills, or destroys comes from the thief, who is Satan.

Sickness and disease have never blessed anybody's life. Rather, they have stolen from people, killed people, and destroyed people's lives. As one preacher said, "Sickness is the foul offspring of its mother, Sin, and its father, Satan."

I want to state emphatically that God is NOT the author of sickness and disease. As Jesus said, He came to give us a life that is filled with abundance—and that includes health and healing.

One reason Jesus came was to reveal the will of God the Father. If we want to know what God is like and to see Him at work, we must look at Jesus. Jesus is the will of God in action. I challenge anyone to find even one place in the gospels where Jesus put sickness or oppression on anybody. In studying the gospels, what we find is that Jesus healed and blessed people everywhere He went.

Acts 10:38 says, "How God anointed Jesus of Nazareth with the Holy Ghost and power: who went about doing good, and healing all that were oppressed of the devil; for God was with him." We see from this passage that Jesus was doing good when He healed people.

We also see that those who were sick were oppressed by the devil. Again, this shows us that sickness is from Satan, and healing is from God. In very simple terms, we can say this: "God is good. And the devil is bad."

Along these same lines, God is not responsible for natural disasters in the earth. The laws governing this earth came into being through the fall of Adam. When Adam sinned, the curse came upon the earth. There was no sickness or disease in the garden of Eden before the fall of man, and there is no sickness in Heaven. There were no natural disasters before the fall of man, and there will be no natural disasters in Heaven.

Because people don't understand this, they often blame God for sickness, accidents, tragedy, and even storms and natural disasters. Insurance policies label these events as "acts of God". However, they are not acts of God. They are acts of the devil.

Jesus never brought any storms on people. Rather, He rebuked the storms. The way some people talk, you would be led to believe that God and the devil had swapped jobs. No, I want to emphasize again that God is always good, and He never contradicts Himself. Jesus would not rebuke something that came from God.

Jesus dealt with sickness the same way He dealt with demons. He rebuked them and commanded them to go. We must follow in the footsteps of Jesus by dealing with sickness like He did. We are to rebuke sickness and command it to leave in Jesus' name. Sickness did not originate with God, and you don't have to put up with it another day!

Day 2

Is Healing God's Will for Me?

Many would agree that God doesn't make people sick, but they wonder if it is always the will of God to heal. We know that Jesus was the will of God in action. I have challenged people to find even one place where Jesus ever told somebody, "I'm sorry, but it's not My will to heal you this time." You will not find Jesus turning any person away who came to Him for healing, and He will not turn you away either! One of the greatest chapters in the New Testament that reveals the nature and will of the Father concerning healing is Matthew chapter 8. Read the following accounts carefully.

> **When He had come down from the mountain, great multitudes followed Him. And behold, a leper came and worshiped Him, saying, "Lord, if You are willing, You can make me clean." Then Jesus put out His hand and touched him, saying, "I am willing; be cleansed." Immediately his leprosy was cleansed. (Matt. 8:1-3)**
>
> **Now when Jesus had entered Capernaum, a centurion came to Him, pleading with Him,**

> **saying, "Lord, my servant is lying at home paralyzed, dreadfully tormented." And Jesus said to him, "I will come and heal him." (Matt. 8:5-7)**
>
> **Now when Jesus had come into Peter's house, He saw his wife's mother lying sick with a fever. So He touched her hand, and the fever left her. And she arose and served them. (Matt. 8:14-15)**
>
> **When evening had come, they brought to Him many who were demon-possessed. And He cast out the spirits with a word, and healed all who were sick, that it might be fulfilled which was spoken by Isaiah the prophet, saying: "He Himself took our infirmities and bore our sicknesses." (Matt. 8:16-17)**

In every one of these situations, Jesus responded with compassion and healing. He did not differentiate between a hopeless leper and Peter's mother-in-law. He healed *all* who were sick in fulfillment of prophecy.

When it comes to the subject of divine healing, one of the greatest difficulties is getting people to see that it is always God's will to heal. Very often, the same people who believe it's not God's will to heal them will spend time and money to seek medical treatment. If they really believe it's not God's will to heal them, why would they try to get out of the will of God by seeking healing through medicine?

Jesus plainly taught through His Words and His actions that sickness and disease come from the enemy, Satan. God wants His children loosed from Satan's bondages!

The following account from Luke illustrates the will of God beautifully:

> **Now He was teaching in one of the synagogues on the Sabbath. And behold, there was a woman who had a spirit of infirmity eighteen years, and was bent over and could in no way raise herself up. But when Jesus saw her, He called her to Him and said to her, "Woman, you are loosed from your infirmity." And He laid His hands on her, and immediately she was made straight, and glorified God.**
>
> **But the ruler of the synagogue answered with indignation, because Jesus had healed on the Sabbath; and he said to the crowd, "There are six days on which men ought to work; therefore come and be healed on them, and not on the Sabbath day."**
>
> **The Lord then answered him and said, "Hypocrite! Does not each one of you on the Sabbath loose his ox or donkey from the stall, and lead it away to water it? So ought not this woman, being a daughter of Abraham, whom Satan has bound—think of it—for eighteen years, be loosed from this bond on the Sabbath?" And when He said these things,**

> **all His adversaries were put to shame; and all the multitude rejoiced for all the glorious things that were done by Him. (Luke 13:10-17)**

This woman had a spirit of infirmity, and notice where it came from: "whom Satan has bound." Jesus also declared that this woman should be loosed and He gave two good reasons why:

1. **Satan had bound her.** God's people should not be bound by sickness or disease. Healing was a promise under the Old Covenant, and Jesus paid the price for our healing under the New Covenant.

2. **She was a daughter of Abraham.** That meant she had a covenant with God. We who are born again also have a covenant with God. The Bible teaches that those who belong to Christ are the seed of Abraham.

   > **And if you are Christ's, then you are Abraham's seed, and heirs according to the promise. (Gal. 3:29)**

If the woman who was a daughter of Abraham ought to be loosed, then New Covenant children of God ought to be loosed! The next time Satan tries to bind you with sickness, you don't have to accept it. You can be healed, because healing is the will of God for you!

Day 3

Forgiveness and Healing Are a Package Deal!

Many have not understood that healing is as much a part of the New Covenant as forgiveness is. Most Christians believe it is always God's will to forgive, but not all believe it is always God's will to heal. Let me show you how God has made forgiveness and healing a package deal!

> **Bless the LORD, O my soul,**
> **And forget not all His benefits:**
> **Who forgives all your iniquities,**
> **Who heals all your diseases. (Ps. 103:2-3)**

Under the Old Covenant, the Lord stated He forgives *all* our iniquities, and heals *all* our diseases. Our covenant today is a new and better covenant. So how could we have less forgiveness or less healing than under the Old Covenant?

Now let's look at what Jesus had to say about this:

> **So He got into a boat, crossed over, and came to His own city. Then behold, they brought to Him a paralytic lying on a bed. When Jesus saw**

> **their faith, He said to the paralytic, "Son, be of good cheer; your sins are forgiven you." And at once some of the scribes said within themselves, "This Man blasphemes!" But Jesus, knowing their thoughts, said, "Why do you think evil in your hearts? For which is easier, to say, 'Your sins are forgiven you,' or to say, 'Arise and walk'? But that you may know that the Son of Man has power on earth to forgive sins"—then He said to the paralytic, "Arise, take up your bed, and go to your house." And he arose and departed to his house. (Matt. 9:1-7)**

Jesus was saying that it is just as easy to receive healing as it is to receive forgiveness. And He proved this by the fact that the paralytic received his forgiveness and healing at the same time. Remember what Psalm 103 says—He forgives *all* our iniquities and He heals *all* our diseases. Healing and forgiveness go hand in hand.

Isaiah 53:4-5 from the Amplified Classic translation says this:

> **Surely He has borne our griefs (sicknesses, weaknesses, and distresses) and carried our sorrows and pains [of punishment], yet we [ignorantly] considered Him stricken, smitten, and afflicted by God [as if with leprosy]. But He was wounded for our transgressions, He was bruised for our guilt and iniquities; the chastisement [needful to obtain] peace and well-being for us was upon Him, and with the stripes [that wounded] Him we are healed and made whole.**

In this passage of Scripture we see the reasons Jesus suffered for us:

1. **He bore our sicknesses and weaknesses for us.**
2. **He bore the punishment of our transgressions (sins).**
3. **He bore our mental anguish.**

The passage closes by stating, "By His stripes we are healed and made whole." Just as much as we are forgiven, we are healed. And to prove that this does not mean spiritual healing, it is repeated in the New Testament in Matthew chapter 8. Here, Jesus healed a leper, a centurion's servant, Peter's mother-in-law, and then all who came to Him that same evening. Immediately following all these healings, it says:

> **When evening had come, they brought to Him many who were demon-possessed. And He cast out the spirits with a word, and healed all who were sick, that it might be fulfilled which was spoken by Isaiah the prophet, saying: "He Himself took our infirmities and bore our sicknesses". (Matt. 8:16-17)**

Jesus healed all these people to fulfill what Isaiah said in Isaiah 53. His healings show that "with the stripes that wounded Him we are healed" does not mean spiritual healing, but rather physical healing.

Here is another very enlightening passage in the New Testament:

> **Is anyone among you sick? Let him call for the elders of the church, and let them pray over him, anointing him with oil in the name of the Lord. And the prayer of faith will save the sick, and the Lord will raise him up. And if he has committed sins, he will be forgiven. (James 5:14-15)**

I love the question, "Is anyone among you sick?" It really implies that there may not be any. And because the early Church understood their covenant of healing, there were not many sick. However, if someone happened to be under attack with sickness, here was the solution: pray over him, anointing him with oil in the name of the Lord. And the prayer of faith will "save" the sick.

The word *save* is translated from the Greek word *sozo*, which means to heal, preserve, save, do well, be whole. So we can rightly interpret that the prayer of faith will *heal* the sick and he will be forgiven! Again, forgiveness and healing go together—a package deal!

I trust you are beginning to see that it is the plan of God for all to be forgiven and to be healed. Isn't it time for you to receive and enjoy your forgiveness and healing?

Day 4

Healing Is the Children's Bread

Let's continue to establish the truth that divine healing belongs to us.

> **And behold, a woman of Canaan came from that region and cried out to Him, saying, "Have mercy on me, O Lord, Son of David! My daughter is severely demon-possessed." But He answered her not a word. And His disciples came and urged Him, saying, "Send her away, for she cries out after us." But He answered and said, "I was not sent except to the lost sheep of the house of Israel." Then she came and worshiped Him, saying, "Lord, help me!" But He answered and said, "It is not good to take *the children's bread* and throw it to the little dogs." And she said, "Yes, Lord, yet even the little dogs eat the crumbs which fall from their masters' table." Then Jesus answered and said to her, "O woman, great is your faith! Let it be to you as you desire." And her daughter was healed from that very hour. (Matt. 15:22-28)**

Notice that Jesus called healing "the children's bread." Who are the children? During the time of this event, the children Jesus referred to were the children of Abraham—God's covenant people. Jesus was saying that healing belonged to the seed of Abraham. This Canaanite woman was not a daughter of Abraham and therefore, did not have a covenant with the God of Israel. However, her faith could see that even a crumb that fell from the children's table would be enough to heal a dog—a non-covenant person.

Throughout history, bread has been a staple of life for mankind. Even the poorest of people had bread to sustain them. How fitting that Jesus would call healing "bread." Bread is for *everyone,* not just a few privileged people. Therefore, we can conclude that healing is for everyone. Jesus paid the price for everyone to be both saved and healed.

In another text, Jesus referred to Himself as the bread of life.

> **"I am the bread of life. Your fathers ate the manna in the wilderness, and are dead. This is the bread which comes down from heaven, that one may eat of it and not die. I am the living bread which came down from heaven. If anyone eats of this bread, he will live forever; and the bread that I shall give is My flesh, which I shall give for the life of the world." (John 6:48-51)**

In the Old Covenant God used many types and shadows of things to come. One of those types was the manna which rained down from Heaven every morning and sustained the children of Israel for forty years in the wilderness. Jesus was saying that people who were spiritually dead, yet in covenant with God, ate supernatural bread in the wilderness to sustain them physically. Now He came down from Heaven to give spiritual life to those who would believe. Spiritual life includes healing and health. Jesus said, "The bread that I shall give is My flesh." Let's look at what the Bible also says about the flesh of Jesus.

> **And the Word became flesh and dwelt among us, and we beheld His glory, the glory as of the only begotten of the Father, full of grace and truth. (John 1:14)**

Jesus *is* the Word of God made flesh. Therefore, if Jesus is the bread of life, the Word of God is the bread of life. As we feed upon the Word of God, we are feeding upon the bread of life.

> **Then Jesus said to them, "Most assuredly, I say to you, unless you eat the flesh of the Son of Man and drink His blood, you have no life in you. Whoever eats My flesh and drinks My blood has eternal life, and I will raise him up at the last day. For My flesh is food indeed, and My blood is drink indeed. He who eats My flesh and drinks My blood abides in Me, and I in him. As the living Father sent Me, and I live because of the Father, so he who feeds on Me will live because of Me." (John 6:53-58)**

Jesus said, "I live because of the Father." He never had a sick day in His life because of the life of the Father in Him. Then Jesus went on to say, "So he who feeds on Me will live because of Me." If we feed on His Word, we can also live free of sickness and disease. Now, lest you think Jesus is endorsing cannibalism, He went on to clarify what He meant.

> **"It is the Spirit who gives life; the flesh profits nothing. The words that I speak to you are spirit, and they are life." (John 6:63)**

Jesus was not saying we must eat His physical flesh and drink His physical blood to have His life. He was saying that His blood will set us free from the power of Satan, and if we feed upon His Word, the Bread of Life, we will have His life and health. After all, healing is the children's bread.

Day 5

Healing Through Prayer

We live in a society that's obsessed with healthcare. You can't even turn on the television without being blasted by multiple drug commercials. And after they finish listing all the potential side effects, you wonder why anyone would take them.

People don't want to be sick! This is obvious by how overused our healthcare system is. And furthermore, God doesn't want people sick either!

> **Beloved, I pray that you may prosper in every way and [that your body] may keep well, even as [I know] your soul keeps well and prospers. (3 John 2 AMPC)**

John was a beloved disciple of Jesus. He knew Jesus well. Under the inspiration of God, he prayed that the bodies of believers would be kept well. Why would John pray for something that wasn't the will of God? He would not. God wants our bodies to be kept well!

Many would ask, "If God wants people well, why are so many sick?" Great question! There are many reasons, but for today we will look at one. Many simply do not understand how to pray scripturally for healing. Prayer is not just throwing a faithless petition up to God. Let's look at what Jesus taught about prayer.

> **Therefore I say to you, whatever things you ask when you pray, believe that you receive them, and you will have them. (Mark 11:24)**

The King James Version states it this way: "Whatsoever things ye desire." This passage is talking about praying for things you desire. For now, we'll just consider one desire: healing for your body. Let's insert the word *healing* into this verse: "When you pray, believe that you receive *healing*, and you will have it."

Some would argue, "But I've prayed before and I didn't receive healing." Many determined their prayer was not answered because of how they felt after praying. However, Jesus said clearly, "And you will have it." I want you to see that first you must *believe* you receive healing.

Many have cried, "But I'm not healed!" That's a person who is going by their head instead of their heart. When you pray, you have to believe you receive healing first, and *then* you will have healing. When are you going to have healing? *After* you believe you receive! When do you believe you receive healing? *Before* you have it!

Some are thinking, *But that doesn't make sense. It's not even common sense!* That's exactly right! It's way above common sense.

Isaiah 55:9 tells us, "For as the heavens are higher than the earth, so are my ways higher than your ways, and my thoughts than your thoughts."

Did it ever occur to you that God's way would be different than your way? This kind of thinking is as high above common sense as the heavens are above the earth. This kind of thinking receives a lot of criticism, but it also receives what it desires from God.

This type of prayer has been working in my life beautifully for over forty years now. One example is when my youngest daughter was just a few months old. She had cold symptoms that developed into a more serious condition with labored breathing. I ended up bringing her to a doctor, and then an emergency room visit. I was told that if there was a third visit, they would diagnose her with asthma. I was determined to receive her healing instead of a negative diagnosis.

I prayed for healing according to Mark 11:24. And then I continued to thank God that my baby was healed, regardless of what I saw and heard. *Faith will stand on what God has said, regardless of what it sees, hears, or feels.* Those symptoms disappeared, but we had several more episodes over the next year that were screaming, "she has asthma." I continued to stand and say only what I believed about it.

We never had to go to the emergency room again, and those symptoms never returned.

Many people fail to receive because they believe the lying symptoms of the devil more than they believe what God has said in His Word. I believe that, as Scripture says, God is not a man that He should lie. If anyone is lying, it's the devil and his symptoms. So when I pray, I believe I receive and refuse to be moved by anything. God is no respecter of persons. You can do the same thing and be assured of victory every time you pray according to the will of God in faith!

Day 6

God's Word Is Medicine

There are many ways to receive healing. However, I believe the most significant method is by simply taking God's Word like you would take medicine.

It is important to understand the life and power that are in the Word of God. He made the world through His words. That reveals how powerful His words really are!

God's Word is a remedy for sickness and disease that never fails. According to the following scriptures, God's Word is full of life, health, and healing.

> **My son, give attention to my words;**
> **Incline your ear to my sayings.**
> **Do not let them depart from your eyes;**
> **Keep them in the midst of your heart;**
> **For they are life to those who find them,**
> **And health to all their flesh. (Prov. 4:20-22)**

The word *health* in verse 22 actually means *medicine* in the original Hebrew text. So we could say that God's Word acts like medicine. God's Word, or God's medicine, will heal *all* your flesh. This means any physical problem you may face is completely curable by the Word of God!

Many will say they believe in healing, but they fail to take God's medicine according to His instructions. Some have never known the instructions, and some simply do not follow the instructions they know. Let's break down God's instructions for taking the medicine, which He prescribes in Proverbs 4:20-22:

1. **Attend to God's Word:** Make it a priority.

2. **Incline your ears unto it:** Listen to His Word every chance you get.

3. **Let it not depart from your eyes:** Look at the healing scriptures and say them out loud repeatedly.

4. **Keep them in the midst of your heart:** This requires meditating day and night, not just once in a while.

All of these instructions imply a continual, ongoing action.

Suppose you were diagnosed with an illness last year and the doctor prescribed a certain medicine. If you get sick with the same illness this year, he will prescribe the same medication again. You wouldn't tell him, "I'm sorry, I can't take that because I already took that medicine last year." We all understand that the same medicine that worked last year will work this year also if we take it again.

It's the same way with God's medicine. In order for it to work for you, you must stay with it and keep taking it every day. Don't have the attitude, "I've already heard those scriptures before," or "I've already tried that." It's through continued meditation on the Word of God that your faith for healing will grow!

There are other parallels between God's medicine and natural medicine. First of all, God's Word is a healing agent just as natural medicine is a healing agent. God's Word contains within it the power to produce healing in our bodies. Psalm 107:20 says, "He sent His *word* and healed them, and delivered them from their destructions."

Second, medicine is no respecter of persons. Medicine doesn't just decide to work for a select few people. The medicine itself contains the ability to bring relief or produce healing. However, God's Word *is* a respecter of faith! His Word works for those who meditate upon it daily. This is how faith for healing comes.

Third and most importantly, medicine must be taken according to directions to be effective. If you take an antibiotic one time a day for two days when the instructions say two times a day for seven days, it will not work for you. It is the same for God's medicine. We must follow the instructions in Proverbs chapter 4. We are to keep His words in the midst of our hearts by continually attending to them.

Notice this: It is only as God's words get in the midst of your heart and stay there that they can produce healing in your body. They must penetrate to your spirit through meditation—attending, hearing, looking, muttering, musing, and pondering—in order to produce healing in your body.

Once God's words penetrate your spirit, they will surely bring health to all your flesh!

Day 7

Speak the Word Only

Death and life are in the power of the tongue,
And those who love it will eat its fruit.

—Proverbs 18:21

So many people are looking for power in their lives. Most fail to realize that they already have power; it is in their tongue—or their words. Our words can bring death, or they can bring life. If we ever fully realize how powerful our words are, we will be far more cautious about what we say.

According to Proverbs chapter 4, God's words are life and health. Therefore it would be wise to speak His Word over our lives. Let's look at the power of the spoken Word of God in a few Bible passages.

Now when Jesus had entered Capernaum, a centurion came to Him, pleading with Him, saying, "Lord, my servant is lying at home paralyzed, dreadfully tormented."

And Jesus said to him, "I will come and heal him."

The centurion answered and said, "Lord, I am not worthy that You should come under my roof. But only speak a word, and my servant will be healed. For I also am a man under authority, having soldiers under me. And I say to this one, 'Go,' and he goes; and to another, 'Come,' and he comes; and to my servant, 'Do this,' and he does it."

When Jesus heard it, He marveled, and said to those who followed, "Assuredly, I say to you, I have not found such great faith, not even in Israel!" (Matt. 8:5-11)

There are only two things that made Jesus marvel—unbelief and great faith. Wouldn't it be terrible to have Jesus marvel at our unbelief? We should always strive to have great faith. Great faith is simply faith in God's Word. It is taking God at His word. God wants us to have the same great faith the centurion had. He wants us to have the same great faith that *He* has! He wants us to have an unshakable confidence in His powerful Word.

There's something else we need to have great confidence in: *our words*! Jesus taught that we must believe in our own words when we speak them if we want them to come to pass.

So Jesus answered and said to them, "Have faith in God. For assuredly, I say to you, whoever says to this mountain, 'Be removed and be cast into the sea,' and does not doubt in his heart, but believes that those things he says will be done, he will have whatever he says." (Mark 11:22-23)

The God kind of faith, or *great faith*, is the kind in which a man believes something with his heart and says what he believes, and it comes to pass. We cannot have great faith apart from speaking *words* of faith. We have been given great and precious promises, and all these promises of God legally belong to us. Healing is a promise to us and therefore belongs to us. But one reason we don't have the reality of all His promises is because we haven't always done our part to believe and speak the promises as we should.

When it comes to sickness, we must understand that it is often determined to stay. Therefore, we have to be more determined to drive it out. This always requires believing and speaking.

Numbers 33:54-55 says,

> **You shall inherit according to the tribes of your fathers. But if you do not drive out the inhabitants of the land from before you, then it shall be that those whom you let remain shall be irritants in your eyes and thorns in your sides, and they shall harass you in the land where you dwell.**

The promised land is a type of our inheritance in Christ. The things we put up with or let remain will be an irritant or a thorn in our sides. If we put up with sickness and disease instead of driving them out by our words, they will be a thorn. If we put up with lack, it will be an irritant. But we can drive these things out of our lives by believing and speaking God's Word.

Joshua chapter 17 tells us the Canaanites were determined to dwell in the land. Joshua told the Israelites they had great power and that they could drive out the Canaanites. We also have great power available to drive out all sickness and disease from our bodies. That power is released by speaking the Word of God only!

Did you know that your words dominate you? God never made a failure; failures are man-made. They are made by wrong believing and wrong speaking.

Our lips can bring healing and health or keep us sick. Our lips can make us victors or failures. We can fill our words with faith or with doubt. We can fill our words with love or with poison.

Our faith will never rise above the words we speak. Wrong thoughts may come and even persist. But if we refuse to put those thoughts into words, they will not become a reality. If we develop the habit of speaking *the Word only*, we can enjoy all the promises God has given us.

Day 8

Redeemed from the Curse

We are going to discuss a word that I believe should get your attention, and that is the word *curse*! Many people think they know what a curse is, and everyone seems to know it's not a good thing. We were taught when we were young that using curse words was very bad, and we often suffered the consequence of using such words.

According to Webster's 1828 Dictionary, to curse is "to utter a wish of evil against one; to imprecate evil upon; to call for mischief or injury to fall upon; to execrate." To imprecate is to invoke against someone or something. To execrate is to feel or express great loathing for someone or something. Many people involved in pagan religions, witchcraft, or Satanism practice placing curses on people as a way of controlling them. Curses are real.

The Bible talks about something called "the curse of the law."

> **Christ has redeemed us from the curse of the law, having become a curse for us (for it is written, "Cursed is everyone who hangs on a tree"), that**

> **the blessing of Abraham might come upon the Gentiles in Christ Jesus, that we might receive the promise of the Spirit through faith. (Gal. 3:13-14)**

If Christ has redeemed us from the curse of the law, what exactly is it? The only way to find out is to go back to the law. The expression "the Law" as found in the New Testament usually refers to the Pentateuch, which are the first five books of the Bible.

When we study these books, we find that the curse or punishment for breaking God's law is threefold:

1. **Poverty**
2. **Sickness**
3. **Spiritual death**

According to Deuteronomy 28, sickness and disease would come upon the people if they failed to observe to do all of God's commandments and His statutes. In this passage, every sickness and disease known to man is called a curse. Let's look at a few of the curses listed.

> **The Lord will smite you with consumption, with fever and inflammation. (Deut. 28:22 AMPC)**

Consumption is pulmonary tuberculosis. And any disease that would cause a fever or inflammation is included in this verse.

> **The Lord will smite you with the boils of Egypt and the tumors, the scurvy and the itch, from which you cannot be healed.**
>
> **The Lord will smite you with madness and blindness and dismay of [mind and] heart. (Deut. 28:27-28 AMPC)**

Boils are infected bumps. Scurvy is a vitamin C deficiency that causes fatigue, swollen bleeding gums, and joint and muscle pain. Madness would be any mental problem (anxiety, depression, etc.).

> **Then the Lord will bring upon you and your descendants extraordinary strokes and blows, great plagues of long continuance, and grievous sicknesses of long duration.**
>
> **Moreover, He will bring upon you all the diseases of Egypt of which you were afraid, and they shall cling to you.**
>
> **Also every sickness and every affliction which is not written in this Book of the Law the Lord will bring upon you until you are destroyed. (Deut. 28:59-61 AMPC)**

I want to bring some clarity to the phrases, "The Lord will smite you" and "the Lord will bring upon you." Dr. Robert Young, a Greek and Hebrew scholar, points out that in the original Hebrew, the verb *will* is in the permissive rather than the causative sense. Actually, it should have been translated, "The Lord *will allow* these plagues to be brought upon you."

God *permits* evil when people move themselves out from His protective covering, but He does not create it.

God does not send plagues and sickness upon His people. Yet He repeatedly warns what will happen if we go against His Word. That's called *mercy*! The devil is just waiting to attack people, and the open door to him is disobedience to the will of God.

Sickness and disease are not the will of God for His people. He does not want a curse to be upon His children due to their disobedience. God wants to bless us with health. That is why He revealed to us in Deuteronomy 28 what would cause blessing and what would cause the curse. Every person on this planet has the freedom of choice. If we are sensible, we will choose the blessing and life.

Since Christ has redeemed us from the curse of the law, then we as believers no longer have the curse in our lives. Many in the body of Christ teach that there are generational curses that believers must be delivered from. I want you to know that no man can curse what God has blessed. All believers in Jesus are legally redeemed from every bit of the curse of the law.

Some may wonder why, then, are so many believers sick? If any believer experiences sickness or disease, it is no longer for the same reason as those who are unsaved. When an unbeliever is in rebellion to God's Word, he has no protection from the curse. The unbeliever is subject to the curse of spiritual death, sickness, and poverty. By contrast, believers have been redeemed and freed from the curse of the law through Christ; they have legal protection from the curse. However, many face difficulties, including sickness, because they *give* place to the devil.

> **Leave no [such] room or foothold for the devil [give no opportunity to him]. (Eph. 4:27 AMPC)**

Some of the ways believers can give place to the devil will be discussed in upcoming days. But for now, I want to mention one way—through a lack of believing the Word of God. Romans 10:17 tells us "faith comes by hearing and hearing by the Word of God." We can school ourselves in faith by continually saying what God says about us.

I want to encourage you to quote these scriptures every day. Simply fill in the blank with the trouble or disease you are facing. *Say:* "According to Deuteronomy 28, __________ is a curse of the law. But according to Galatians 3:13, Christ has redeemed me from the curse of the law. Therefore, I no longer have __________."

As you continue to confess this, you will find that the symptoms and troubles will begin to disappear.

Day 9

Discerning the Lord's Body

After Adam and Eve sinned, the curse came upon the human race. As we saw yesterday, a description of the curse can be found in the book of Deuteronomy. The curse includes every sickness and disease. But thank God, according to Galatians 3:13, Christ has redeemed us from the curse by being made a curse for us.

In Galatians 3:29, believers in Jesus are called the seed of Abraham. Because Jesus took the curse, the blessing of Abraham has come upon us. The blessing includes healing from every sickness and every disease.

Now, if you've been a Christian for any length of time, you have noticed that plenty of Christians suffer with sickness and disease. So is Galatians 3:13 a contradiction? Absolutely not! If a born again believer is suffering with sickness and disease, it is definitely not the will of God, and the answer has decisively been given through the shed blood of Jesus.

You may be asking, "So why, then, are believers suffering with sickness and disease?" It is not for the same reasons as those who do not belong to Jesus. Those who are unsaved have not been redeemed from the curse of the law. But if a believer has sickness and disease in their body, there is a cause other than the curse.

> **Leave no [such] room or foothold for the devil [give no opportunity to him]. (Eph. 4:27 AMPC)**

We are commanded to give no place or opportunity to the devil. How can we as believers give the devil a place in us? Here's a good starting place for us today:

> **Therefore whoever eats this bread or drinks this cup of the Lord in an unworthy manner will be guilty of the body and blood of the Lord. *But let a man examine himself,* and so let him eat of the bread and drink of the cup. For he who eats and drinks in an unworthy manner eats and drinks judgment to himself, *not discerning the Lord's body.* For this reason many are weak and sick among you, and many sleep. For if we would judge ourselves, we would not be judged. But when we are judged, we are chastened by the Lord, that we may not be condemned with the world. (1 Cor. 11:27-32, emphasis mine)**

The word *sleep* in this passage is the same Greek word that Jesus used when saying Lazarus is sleeping. It actually means *decease* or *be dead.* So we see that believers can be weak, sick, or die prematurely by not discerning the Lord's body. How do we discern the Lord's body?

Discerning the Lord's body has a two-fold application.

1. **Discerning Jesus' physical body**
   According to 1 Peter 2:24, "by whose stripes you were healed," Jesus took a beating so that we could receive healing.

We must always remember that healing has been provided for us, as we discussed in prior days. If we don't remember His benefits, we will not enjoy His benefits. Psalm 103 says, "forget not all His benefits."

2. **Discerning Jesus' spiritual body**
   Jesus is the Head and the Church is His body. Christians must recognize how their actions will affect others in the body, or it could lead to weakness, sickness, and premature death. In the book of Ephesians, we see how the body is supposed to function:

> **For because of Him the whole body (the church, in all its various parts), closely joined and firmly knit together by the joints and ligaments with which it is supplied, *when each part [with power adapted to its need] is working properly [in all its functions], grows to full maturity, building itself up in love.* (Eph 4:16 AMPC, emphasis mine)**

There is a supply for every member to bring to the body. We must discern how our supply is affecting the body. Are we helping to build up the body or are we contributing to making it less effective? Many believers have never given much thought to the truth that we must be right about how we treat other believers. If we are not bringing our supply to the body, it will hurt the other believers in some measure.

One of the most important places to consider this is in the local church. God is the One who instituted local churches and put pastors over them to teach, guide, and protect the sheep. The way we treat our local church will have a definite effect on our health. Having been pastors for over forty years, my husband and I have observed that when believers do not have a local church, or they do not treat the members properly, those believers suffer needlessly.

Here are four steps to properly discern the local church:

1. **Attend services.**
   First of all, we must recognize that we need a local church and should find the one God is calling us to and attend it regularly.

2. **Pray for the pastor and the church.**
   Your pastor and fellow church members are all facing the same demonic opposition as you, and they need your prayers.

3. **Give financially to your local church.**
   Withholding finances from your local church hinders the supply that other people could receive from your church's ministry.

4. **Serve in the ministry of helps.**
   It is important that you not only attend services but get involved in helping so the local body can grow together.

We realize there are exceptions where a believer cannot be a part of a local church. But for the vast majority, the plan of God is always that sheep be part of a group and not loners in danger of wolves.

Remember, the apostle Paul said, "For this reason, *many* are weak, sick, and die prematurely, *not discerning the Lord's body.*" This is a good starting point for examining our lives. If we will discern our proper supply in the local church, we should never be weak, sick, or die prematurely.

Day 10

Walk in Love and Live Healed - Part 1

If I were suffering from sickness and disease, even after praying for healing, I would want to know why! For the past few days, we have been talking about the truth that Christians are redeemed from the curse of sickness and disease, but they can still open a door to the devil that allows sickness to come upon them. There are reasons why believers suffer sickness, and we saw a key scriptural passage that brings this truth out.

> **Therefore whoever eats this bread or drinks this cup of the Lord in an unworthy manner will be guilty of the body and blood of the Lord. But let a man examine himself, and so let him eat of the bread and drink of the cup. For he who eats and drinks in an unworthy manner eats and drinks judgment to himself, not discerning the Lord's body. For this reason many are weak and sick among you, and many sleep. (1 Cor. 11:27-30)**

The way we receive communion will affect our health. Not properly discerning the Lord's body is the reason many are weak and sick, and many die prematurely.

We looked at the two applications of this:

1. **Discerning Jesus' physical body.**
2. **Discerning Jesus' spiritual body.**

Before we receive communion, we are supposed to examine ourselves. If I were suffering with sickness and disease that was stubbornly hanging on, the first place I would examine is my love walk. How am I treating other people?

A lot of people have the erroneous idea that what they do is between them and God, and nobody else's business. This is simply not true. Whether you are a believer in Jesus Christ or not, the decisions you make for your life affect other people—especially your children.

Regarding your children, Exodus 34:6-7 says:

> **"The LORD, the LORD God, merciful and gracious, longsuffering, and abounding in goodness and truth, keeping mercy for thousands, forgiving iniquity and transgression and sin, by no means clearing the guilty, visiting the iniquity of the fathers upon the children and the children's children to the third and the fourth generation."**

God is so merciful. But if we persist in living in sin, it will have a negative effect, not only on us and our children but also on future generations, until someone surrenders to the Lord and turns that train around. Decisions we make and lifestyles we live influence and affect the thinking and outcome of our children. In the same way, what we do affects other believers in the church.

> **From whom the whole body, joined and knit together by what every joint *supplies*, according to the effective working by which every part does its share, causes growth of the body for the edifying of itself in love. (Eph. 4:16, emphasis mine)**

When we become a member of the body of Christ, and particularly of a local church, the Bible says we become joined and knit together. What you are joined to will be affected by what you do. We should always be asking ourselves, *How is this action I'm about to take going to affect those around me?* If it will cause injury, then you shouldn't do it.

If only people understood how much walking in love is connected to their receiving healing! It may only be a very small adjustment that's needed for them to be free of sickness and pain.

One very important area to examine is whether we have forgiven someone who we feel has wronged us. There's a story of a Christian woman who was faithfully involved in her local church, yet had suffered from stomach trouble and respiratory problems for a long time. After hearing a guest speaker teach about the importance of love and forgiveness, she realized what her problem was. She had fought with her brother, who was also a Christian, and they had not even spoken to each other in twenty-five years. She decided it was time to call him and ask for forgiveness. After she did, she lay down to take a nap before the evening service. When she woke up, she realized she was completely healed of all her symptoms!

Notice it didn't require a minister laying hands upon her to receive her healing. All along, it was a lack of walking in love that hindered her from good health. When you refuse to forgive someone, whether they were wrong or you just think they were wrong, you open the door to Satan to attack your body physically.

First Corinthians 13:5 from the Amplified Classic translation says, "Love pays no attention to a suffered wrong." Many people would never have to get into a healing line if they would just walk in love and forgiveness with others. If you've been in prayer lines, especially with ministers who are well known for the healing anointing, and nothing physically has changed, it would be a good idea to start examining yourself to see if you're walking in love.

There is a story of another woman who had a bad habit of speaking against the members of her local church. One day, she was diagnosed with terminal cancer and she was at death's doorstep. When the pastor and some of the members came to her house to pray for her, she said, "Before you pray, I need to ask for forgiveness from all of you. For years, I have sown cancer into the church through my words, and now I have reaped cancer as a result." She repented, and when the pastor and members prayed for her, she was instantly healed of cancer.

One of Jesus' greatest teachings on faith and prayer reveals the importance of forgiveness.

> **"Therefore I say to you, whatever things you ask when you pray, believe that you receive them, and you will have them.**
>
> **And whenever you stand praying, if you have anything against anyone, forgive him, that your Father in heaven may also forgive you your trespasses. But if you do not forgive, neither will your Father in heaven forgive your trespasses." (Mark 11:24-26)**

You cannot receive answered prayer if you have unforgiveness toward anybody for any reason! Answered prayer includes healing of sickness and disease. Jesus also taught us to pray, "Forgive us our trespasses, *as* we forgive those who trespass against us." If we are quick to forgive others, and quick to receive forgiveness, we will be quick to receive healing.

Day 11

Walk in Love and Live Healed - Part 2

We have seen that although Christians are redeemed from the curse of sickness and disease, they can still open a door to the devil that allows sickness to come upon them. First Corinthians chapter 11 reveals that many are weak, sick, and die prematurely because they have not properly discerned the Lord's body.

Part of discerning the Lord's body is understanding that what we do has an effect on those around us, positive or negative. As we mentioned yesterday, one of the greatest areas to guard is our mouth. Always ask yourself, *How is what I am about to say going to affect the other person? Is what I'm about to say going to bring edification or destruction?* Sometimes we get to talking about something another person has said or done, and they could have already repented of it. If the Lord has forgiven them, He has forgotten it. If we bring it up again, we violate the law of love.

Did you know that walking in love is a *royal law*?

> **If you really fulfill the royal law according to the Scripture, "You shall love your neighbor as yourself," you do well. (James 2:8)**

Loving your neighbor as yourself is the *royal law* of love. Would you want someone to talk about you the way you are talking about them? Would you want someone to treat you the way you are treating them? Let's take this a step further: Would you say it or do it to Jesus? If we are His body, then when we mistreat a member of the body, we are mistreating Jesus. Jesus made this clear when speaking to Saul of Tarsus:

> **Then he fell to the ground, and heard a voice saying to him, "Saul, Saul, why are you persecuting Me?" And he said, "Who are You, Lord?" Then the Lord said, "I am Jesus, whom you are persecuting." (Acts 9:4-5)**

Saul was arresting and killing Christians, but Jesus said Saul was persecuting Him. So we can see that how we treat the body is part of discerning the Lord's body. If I love my fellow church members, I will be careful to share the load in serving at church so that another is not overburdened. If I love my fellow church members, I will be careful about what I say about them, and I will pray for them. If I love my fellow church members, I will be mindful about my giving so that the whole church can accomplish its mission. We must discern that we are not an island, and selfishness has no place in the church of the Lord Jesus Christ.

One of the reasons we see more sickness in the church today is that more people are slandering and hurting others than in the past. They have been influenced by the spirit of the world. Bitterness and unforgiveness have a high price tag. We must ask ourselves if we can afford to have strife, bitterness, and unforgiveness in our lives. The answer is, Not if we want to live healed! Does what you're about to say meet the criteria of Philippians 4:8 below?

> **Finally, brethren, whatever things are true, whatever things are noble, whatever things are just, whatever things are pure, whatever things are lovely, whatever things are of good report, if there is any virtue and if there is anything praiseworthy—meditate on these things.**

Some things could be true, but they are not lovely. Some things are true, but they are not pure. Let's practice the law of love, and live the healed life that Jesus paid for us to have!

Day 12

Walk in Love and Live Healed - Part 3

Over the past few days we have studied these twin truths: Christ has redeemed us from sickness and disease, yet we can open a door to the enemy, who brings the very curse we're redeemed from. How do we keep the door shut and sickness out? As the apostle Paul explains, if we want to avoid becoming weak and sick we must properly discern the body of Christ.

One aspect of discerning the Lord's body is walking in love with other people. If your faith is going to work and be effective, you will have to put the God kind of love to work. *God's love is the only thing that's going to win out in the end because it NEVER FAILS.*

Galatians 5:6 says,

> **For in Christ Jesus neither circumcision nor uncircumcision avails anything, but faith working through love.**

It takes faith to receive God's healing. Since faith works by love, we also need to let the love of God rule our words and actions. In order to let love rule, we need to know exactly what the love of God is.

Many think love is a feeling. We will certainly have feelings throughout our lives. However, as we will see, every description of the God kind of love is an action, and not a feeling. One of the reasons the divorce rate is so high is because many have lost their romantic feelings, which they assume is love. If we would live by God's definition of love, we would never fail in our marriages. Likewise, if we would walk in God's love, we would never fail to receive our healing. Let's take a look at the description of the God kind of love.

> **Love endures long and is patient and kind; love never is envious nor boils over with jealousy, is not boastful or vainglorious, does not display itself haughtily.**
>
> **It is not conceited (arrogant and inflated with pride); it is not rude (unmannerly) and does not act unbecomingly. Love (God's love in us) does not insist on its own rights or its own way, for it is not self-seeking; it is not touchy or fretful or resentful; it takes no account of the evil done to it [it pays no attention to a suffered wrong].**
>
> **It does not rejoice at injustice and unrighteousness, but rejoices when right and truth prevail.**

> **Love bears up under anything and everything that comes, is ever ready to believe the best of every person, its hopes are fadeless under all circumstances, and it endures everything [without weakening].**
>
> **Love never fails [never fades out or becomes obsolete or comes to an end]. (1 Cor. 13:4-8 AMPC)**

Believers need to understand how much ill will and animosity will harm them. It can affect your spiritual growth, can cause your prayers to be hindered, and open the door to sickness. It can even shorten your life. Why? Every step out of love is a step into sin. And sin destroys. If you realize you have gotten away from walking in love, get back to it as fast as you can. Then you can live under God's abundant provision and promises and enjoy His great blessings in your life!

Did you know that love is not a suggestion? It is a commandment. God wouldn't command us to do something we weren't able to do. He has given us *His* love to use, and we *are able* to walk in love.

1 John 4:20-21 says,

> **If someone says, "I love God," and hates his brother, he is a liar; for he who does not love his brother whom he has seen, how can he love God whom he has not seen? And this commandment we have from Him: that he who loves God must love his brother also.**

I would venture to say that if I asked you today, "Do you love God?", your answer would be overwhelmingly, "YES!" But an equally important question is: Are you walking in love with others? Do you love your husband or wife? Do you love your children? Your brother or sister in Christ? Your neighbors?

Husbands, when was the last time you woke up early on your day off and made breakfast for your wife and children? When was the last time you asked your wife if there was something you could do to help her, instead of taking off and doing what you wanted to do?

Wives, when was the last time you did something nice for your husband or children without complaining and letting them know it was a sacrifice? Husbands and wives, when was the last time you said, "I love you" to one another in a kind and tender way?

Love is an attitude and an action, not a feeling. Just like faith is expressed through actions, love must be expressed through actions. Just as faith is expressed by your words, *love* is expressed by words.

We express our love by saying, "I love you" and by acting lovingly toward others. The more you say "I love you" and other endearing words to one another, and the more you practice actions of love, the more you will develop that love and the easier it will become.

Every Christian must decide for himself what he would like more:

Health or sickness?
Joy or sorrow?
Provision or poverty?

If you want to receive healing, live in divine health, and fulfill the number of your days, you will have to choose to walk in love. Today is a great day to start walking in love and receive your healing!

Day 13

Hung by the Tongue

There are many reasons why believers fail to receive divine healing. One of those reasons is two inches below their nose.

> **For He who would love life**
> **And see good days,**
> **Let him refrain his tongue from evil,**
> **And his lips from speaking deceit. (1 Pet. 3:10)**

If you want to love your life and see good days, you must learn to *master your tongue*. In other words, control what you say! This includes refraining from speaking evil of other people. It also includes refraining from speaking against your healing. You cannot expect to receive anything from God if you continually disagree with Him.

Proverbs 18:21 tells us, *"Death and life are in the power of the tongue, and those who love it will eat its fruit."* The Message Bible says it this way: "*Words kill, words give life; they're either poison or fruit—you choose.*" God has given man the power of words. Many people have no idea how powerful their words are. But words can kill or give life.

When it comes to our health and well-being, it is never beneficial to speak negatively about it. The more we talk about the problem, the worse it will become. This seems to be the opposite of what we see and hear in our world today. Professionals everywhere encourage people to talk about the problems. We have many talk shows where people publicly talk about their personal problems. What we need are more programs that talk about the answers, like the ones from Miller Ministries!

Jesus had something to say about our words.

> **"For assuredly, I say to you, whoever says to this mountain, 'Be removed and be cast into the sea,' and does not doubt in his heart, but believes that those things he says will be done, he will have whatever he says." (Mark 11:23)**

Jesus never told a lie. He said that the things we say with our mouths and believe in our hearts are exactly what we will have. A mountain represents a problem we are facing in life, for example, a sickness or disease. Jesus told us to say something to the mountain: "BE REMOVED!"

So many people are talking *about* the mountains in their lives instead of talking *to* the mountains. And that is why the sickness and disease are still in their bodies. We could say, they are hung by their tongue!

It's the easiest thing in the world to just talk about the sickness or disease you are dealing with. Most people talk about their health issues, as if that will console them somehow. But according to Jesus, *what you say and believe is what you get*. That is the same as saying death and life are in the power of the tongue.

> **So then faith comes by hearing, and hearing by the word of God. (Rom. 10:17)**

Since faith comes by hearing, the more you hear something, the more you'll believe it. Therefore, the more you say it, the more you hear it, and the more you believe it. We have actually been created by God to live our lives by our words.

Genesis says we are made in the likeness of God. This is the same way that God operates. He spoke, and then things came into existence. Whether we like it or not, the Bible makes it clear that *everything we have today in life is the sum total of what we've believed in our hearts and spoken with our mouths.*

Romans 10:9-10 says, "that if you confess with your mouth the Lord Jesus and believe in your heart that God has raised Him from the dead, you will be saved. For with the heart one believes unto righteousness, and with the mouth confession is made unto salvation." The original Greek word translated as *salvation* actually means to heal, preserve, save, and make whole. So we could translate the last part of verse 10 like this: "...and with the mouth confession is made unto health and wholeness."

Words always have something to do with our receiving from God. Proverbs 12:18 from the Amplified Classic translation says, "There are those who speak rashly, like the piercing of a sword, but the tongue of the wise brings healing."

The whole world is programmed to be negative. If we spend too much time around negative people, we will be negative. You do not want to think like the world thinks when it comes to disease. You want to think and speak healing words so you can live healed. As you spend time daily meditating upon healing scriptures, you will find it easier to *speak the word only*. Then you will find that instead of being hung by your tongue, you will be healed by your tongue!

Day 14

Hold Fast to God's Word

A very important truth to understand is that anything God blesses us with, the devil will try to steal.

> **The thief does not come except to steal, and to kill, and to destroy. I have come that they may have life, and that they may have it more abundantly. (John 10:10)**

You can love the Lord, serve Him faithfully, and still struggle with sickness and pain. We have an enemy that does not want us to enjoy our benefit of healing. He will try everything to keep us from walking in health and victory. No matter how much he tries, though, we have a greater weapon, and that is the Word of God. Therefore, we must be committed to staying full of the Word of God and holding fast to it in times of trouble.

Perhaps you have received healing for your body in the past, but then that sickness came back on you. Why? Because the devil will always try to gain entrance again in the place he once occupied. Here is how the Lord Jesus explained it:

> **When an unclean spirit goes out of a man, he goes through dry places, seeking rest, and finds none. Then he says, 'I will return to my house from which I came.' And when he comes, he finds it empty, swept, and put in order. Then he goes and takes with him seven other spirits more wicked than himself, and they enter and dwell there; and the last state of that man is worse than the first. So shall it also be with this wicked generation. (Matt. 12:43-45)**

This passage shows us the devil's persistence. If the devil returns with symptoms of sickness or disease, we do not want him to find us empty. That means we don't want him to find a weak spirit because we have not been putting the Word of God into it continually.

We all know that it can be a challenge to keep our hearts full of God's Word—everyone must contend with the busyness of life. Not only that, our enemy the devil will put extra pressure on us to keep us from spending time in the Word of God. He knows that is where our answers lie. You see, when you spend time meditating upon God's Word, faith comes. It takes faith to receive your healing and it takes faith to keep your healing.

First Timothy 6:12 tells us to "fight the good fight of faith". Faith always has a fight with it because we live in this fallen world, which is Satan's territory. The good news is that the victory over him has already been won. Our fight isn't to win the victory, but rather to receive and keep that victory.

Some may have thought, "If God really healed me, then I would always stay healed." Yes, God really heals, but we still have to maintain our healing by our *faith*.

Jesus said, "But hold fast what you have till I come" (Rev. 2:25).

If we are told to hold fast to what we have, this means it's possible to let go of it—and lose it. In order to hold fast, we must continually exercise our faith for healing. This means that daily we are meditating upon healing scriptures and daily we are releasing our faith by our words. That's how we live healed.

Peter instructs us to live in resistance mode against the devil:

> **Be sober, be vigilant; because your adversary the devil walks about like a roaring lion, seeking whom he may devour. Resist him, steadfast in the faith. (1 Pet. 5:8-9)**

It's good to know that our answer is to resist the devil. But how exactly do we do that?

1. **We make a decision that we will not be moved by what we see or feel.**

   > **NOW FAITH is the assurance (the confirmation, the title deed) of the things [we] hope for, being the proof of things [we] do not see and the conviction of their reality [faith perceiving as real fact what is not revealed to the senses]. (Heb. 11:1 AMPC)**

There are times when you must stand on what God says, believing it regardless of how you feel or what the natural circumstances look like. Meditating upon the Word of God will help you to see that you are already healed instead of being discouraged by a bad report.

2. **We must continue to say only what God says about the situation.**

   Let us hold fast the profession of our faith without wavering; (for he is faithful that promised.) (Heb. 10:23 KJV)

It is so vital to only say what God says in His Word in order to receive and keep our healing. We cannot speak God's Word one day, talk about sickness or pain the next, and expect to be healed.

There have been times when I go to walk my dog, and my knee will try to hurt and stop me. My trained reaction is always, "Oh no you don't! I refuse to have knee pain. My youth is renewed like the eagle's and I am completely healed by the stripes of Jesus!" I continue to walk as an act of faith, and the pain disappears. If I were to say, "Oh no, I guess I can't walk now. I thought I was healed," I would not be holding fast to my healing.

Jesus already defeated the devil and purchased our healing for us. We have been given authority over all the power the devil. I encourage you to exercise that authority by holding fast to your healing and by resisting the devil's sickness, disease, and pain every day of your life.

Day 15

Worry Is a Deadly Habit

Beloved, I pray that you may prosper in all things and be in health, just as your soul prospers.

—3 John 2

God wants us to have a good life, a life that prospers in every area. We all know that a sick life does not fulfill the definition of a prosperous life. God has provided healing for every one of us, but it will show up in our lives according to the measure that our soul prospers. When do our souls prosper? When we embrace God's thoughts! So, the more we embrace His thoughts, the more prosperous our souls will be. And as our souls prosper, so does our healing and health.

One thing that will rob your soul of being prosperous is worry. Why? Because when we worry, we can't embrace God's thoughts. Worry can very quickly sabotage your healing. Worry is the opposite of faith. Worry is believing the worst instead of the best. *Worry is fear.* Worrying about your health is a great big invitation to the devil to put sickness and disease on you. This is one of the problems Job had. He had a worry problem.

> **For the thing which I greatly feared is come upon me, and that which I was afraid of is come unto me. (Job 3:25 KJV)**

Job's fear left a wide open door to the devil to attack him, and not just in health, but in almost every arena of his life.

Jesus actually taught us not to worry:

> **"Therefore I say to you, do not worry about your life... Which of you by worrying can add one cubit to his stature?" (Matt. 6:25,27)**

If you can't add one inch to your height or one hair to your head by worrying, then you absolutely cannot change more serious situations in your life by worrying. Medical science tells us that smoking and drinking are habits that can ruin your health and send you to an early grave. But did you know that worry will destroy your health and kill you even faster than smoking and drinking? Jesus was so serious about us not worrying that He commanded us not to do it. If we ignore His commandments, that is a form of sin because it is unbelief. Most Christians would agree that stealing, lying, and murder are sins, but they don't realize that worry—because it is unbelief—is also a sin.

I think we all know it's not good to worry, but most people are so highly developed in their worry skills that they don't even realize how much they worry to begin with. To worry is to meditate in the negative direction. The mind is not built to handle worry, so those who worry will eventually have a breakdown, first of the mind and then the body. Worry cannot receive healing; it can only receive sickness.

So how can we stop this deadly worry habit and enjoy good health?

> **Casting all your care upon Him, for He cares for you. (1 Pet. 5:7)**

The Amplified Classic translation says it this way:

> **Casting the whole of your care [all your anxieties, all your worries, all your concerns, once and for all] on Him, for He cares for you affectionately and cares about you watchfully.**

You are to give your worries to Jesus and leave them there. As long as you are worrying about something, all the prayer in the world won't change it! By casting the care completely over on the Lord, you are demonstrating that you trust Him to answer your prayer.

When we really trust that He will do what He says in His Word, then there will be no room left for worry and fear.

Trust means *faith*. Faith is how we obtain promises, not by worry.

Here is a glimpse of what faith will do:

> **Who through faith subdued kingdoms, worked righteousness, obtained promises, stopped the mouths of lions, quenched the violence of fire, escaped the edge of the sword, out of weakness were made strong, became valiant in battle, turned to flight the armies of the aliens. Women received their dead raised to life again. (Heb. 11:33-35)**

But worry has the opposite effect. No promises will be obtained if you remain in a state of worry. And that is why as long as you are worrying, you will not receive healing or anything else from the Lord.

There is a story in the Bible of a woman who had an issue of blood for twelve long years. We learn an important lesson about healing from her story. After she was healed, Jesus told her to go in peace.

> **And He said to her, Daughter, your faith (your trust and confidence in Me, springing from faith in God) has restored you to health. Go in (into) peace and be continually healed and freed from your [distressing bodily] disease. (Mark 5:34 AMPC)**

Jesus understood that in order for this woman to keep her healing, she had to stay in peace and not worry. The same is true for you and me today. We are to cast all our cares upon the Lord and trust Him to do exactly what He said He would do in His Word.

Here is another scriptural admonition not to worry.

> **Do not fret or have any anxiety about anything, but in every circumstance and in everything, by prayer and petition (definite requests), with thanksgiving, continue to make your wants known to God.**
>
> **And God's peace [shall be yours, that tranquil state of a soul assured of its salvation through Christ, and so fearing nothing from God and being content with its earthly lot of whatever sort that is, that peace] which transcends all understanding shall garrison and mount guard over your hearts and minds in Christ Jesus. (Phil. 4:6-7 AMPC)**

The next time you catch yourself starting to worry about something, declare that you refuse to worry. Pray and ask the Lord for the answer you need. Then give Him thanksgiving and praise because the answer is on the way.

Day 16

Hear and Be Healed

When it comes to divine healing, it is so important to understand that it is always received by faith. Healing always manifests because of the faith of someone—whether it's the preacher, the one who is sick, or a loved one standing in the gap. I have preferred to use my own faith because then I can be assured that someone is believing!

If you have need of faith, the Bible teaches you how to get it. "Faith comes by hearing, and hearing by the Word of God" (Rom. 10:17).

When the Bible talks about hearing in reference to faith, it is always referring to hearing with your spiritual ears, not just your physical ears. Many people throughout history have heard the sayings of Jesus with their physical ears, yet have not understood and received them. In order to benefit from the sayings of Jesus, you must hear them with your spiritual ears and believe them with your spirit. Jesus frequently told His listeners, "He who has ears to hear, let him hear!" When He spoke these words, He was referring to our spiritual ears.

We also see this from several passages, including Luke 5:15: "And great multitudes came together to hear, and to be healed by Him of their infirmities." I think that many people have this idea that Jesus just went everywhere healing everybody He came in contact with. But if you read the gospels carefully, you find that this is simply not true. Jesus knew that if the people did not hear His sayings with their spiritual understanding, they could not receive healing.

Hearing with our spiritual ears begins with hearing Jesus' words. The gospels are full of examples of Him teaching, preaching, and healing. But let's note the order of these three: teaching comes first. Why? Because unless the people hear the good news, they have nothing to attach their faith to, and they will not be able to receive healing. We see just one of many examples of this order in Matthew 9:35:

> **Then Jesus went about all the cities and villages, teaching in their synagogues, preaching the gospel of the kingdom, and healing every sickness and every disease among the people.**

We see that Jesus placed teaching first, preaching second, and healing last. Of course, many people want to reverse the order. They would prefer to run to a meeting and have someone heal them without spending any quality time hearing.

Those who would not hear Jesus during His earthly ministry did not receive healing. Again, this is referring to hearing with your spiritual ears, because in Nazareth the people certainly heard with their physical ears. However, very few people were healed there.

Here is the account in Mark chapter 6:

> **And when the Sabbath had come, He began to teach in the synagogue. And many hearing Him were astonished, saying, "Where did this Man get these things? And what wisdom is this which is given to Him, that such mighty works are performed by His hands! Is this not the carpenter, the Son of Mary, and brother of James, Joses, Judas, and Simon? And are not His sisters here with us?" So they were offended at Him.**
>
> **But Jesus said to them, "A prophet is not without honor except in his own country, among his own relatives, and in his own house." Now He could do no mighty work there, except that He laid His hands on a few sick people and healed them. And He marveled because of their unbelief. Then He went about the villages in a circuit, *teaching*.**

Since faith comes by hearing the Word of God, the cure for their unbelief was teaching. Even though Jesus was the Son of God, and divine blood flowed through His veins, He still could not heal people who were full of unbelief. God does not override our unbelief! Faith is required, and if people refuse to believe, they will have to live without their healing.

What kept the people from hearing and receiving? *Unbelief.* Why did they refuse to believe? *Familiarity.* The more familiar we are with someone, the harder it can be to receive from them. We simply see them as a regular person instead of someone anointed by the Holy Spirit to help us.

Now let's see what the people who came to Jesus actually heard:

> **"The Spirit of the LORD is upon Me,**
> **Because He has anointed Me**
> ***To preach* the gospel to the poor;**
> **He has sent Me *to heal* the brokenhearted,**
> **To proclaim liberty to the captives**
> **And recovery of sight to the blind,**
> ***To set at liberty* those who are oppressed;**
> **To proclaim the acceptable year of the LORD."**
> **(Luke 4:18-19, emphasis mine)**

Luke 5:15 says, "great multitudes came together to hear, and to be healed by Him of their infirmities." They heard Jesus say He came to heal, to give recovery of sight to the blind, and to set at liberty those who were oppressed. Was this effective? YES! The woman with the issue of blood was healed because of what she heard.

> **Now a certain woman had a flow of blood for twelve years, and had suffered many things from many physicians. She had spent all that she had and was no better, but rather grew worse. *When she heard about Jesus*, she came behind Him in the crowd and touched His garment. For she**

> **said, "If only I may touch His clothes, I shall be made well."**
>
> **Immediately the fountain of her blood was dried up, and she felt in her body that she was healed of the affliction. (Mark 5:25-29, emphasis mine)**

This woman heard truth with both her natural and her spiritual ears. Then, having heard and received the truth, she acted upon it. Today, you have had the opportunity to hear truth. Now I encourage you to continue hearing and hearing with your spiritual ears until your faith is ready to receive healing.

Day 17

God Keeps His Promises

How can you be sure that God will heal you every time you need it? You have His Word on it! Do you believe it is God's will to keep His promises? Here are a few promises of God regarding healing:

> **For I am the LORD who heals you. (Exod. 15:26)**
>
> **He Himself took our infirmities**
> **And bore our sicknesses. (Matt. 8:17)**
>
> **Who Himself bore our sins in His own body on the tree, that we, having died to sins, might live for righteousness—by whose stripes you were healed. (1 Pet. 2:24)**

All these promises are for YOU! They are not for a few highly favored people. And since God said it in His Word, you can believe it!

Even though healing is for all, it must be received by *faith*, or we could say by *trust*. Therefore, before anyone can have steadfast faith for healing, they must be rid of all uncertainty about God's will to heal. God's promises are a revelation of what God is eager to do for us. Until we know the promises that pertain to our situation, there is nothing on which to base our faith.

The Bible teaches us that faith comes by hearing, and hearing what the Word of God promises. Faith is simply expecting God to do what He promised to do. Faith is believing that God's words are true.

> **God is not a man, that He should lie,**
> **Nor a son of man, that He should repent.**
> **Has He said, and will He not do?**
> **Or has He spoken, and will He not make it good?**
> **(Num. 23:19)**

If someone you trusted promised to give you $1,000 tomorrow, and they were in the habit of keeping their word, you would believe and act like it was true. Shouldn't we trust our Heavenly Father more than we trust the word of any man?

Regarding healing, there are only two positions a person can have: belief or unbelief. Either the Word of God is true, or it is not. God is either reliable, or He is not. Will we believe the Word of God is truthful, or not?

Genuine faith in God and in His Word will step out on what He has said, regardless of what we see, feel, or sense in the natural realm. Faith is a decisive act that depends only upon God's Word. Faith ignores every natural symptom or evidence which is contrary to what God's Word says.

One of my favorite definitions of faith is found in Hebrews.

> **NOW FAITH is the assurance (the confirmation, the title deed) of the things [we] hope for, being the proof of things [we] do not see and the conviction of their reality [faith perceiving as real fact what is not revealed to the senses]. (Heb. 11:1 AMPC)**

Genuine faith will count healing as a real fact, *even if your body says you are not healed.* As Christians, one of the most important lessons we must learn is to not be moved by circumstances that contradict the Word of God. We must also learn to be patient and not get discouraged if things don't change immediately.

The devil doesn't let anybody have a free pass. He will endeavor to deceive you so you will give up before you see the manifestation. However, if you will not be moved by what you feel and see, and stand firm on what God says, you will win the battle every time!

I heard the story of a lady from New York, who many years ago was on her deathbed being ravaged by the effects of tuberculosis. She was a wonderful Christian, but had never heard about divine healing. One afternoon she was reading the Bible and came across 1 Peter 2:24,

> **"Who Himself bore our sins in His own body on the tree, that we, having died to sins, might live for righteousness..."**

As she read this verse, she began to weep with gratitude for the salvation Jesus had provided for her. She knew when this disease had run its course, she would be ready to die and go to Heaven. Then she decided to read further: **"...by whose stripes you were healed."**

She looked back and noticed that Jesus had already bore her sins. It was in the past. It was real to her, and nobody could make her doubt it. But what about the rest of the verse? Could it be true? Did it mean what it said? She concluded that it must be true.

She cried out, "Mother, did you know that God has said in His Word that I was healed? I never saw this before. It's already done. I am healed. Get my clothes and bring them here!"

Her mother tried to calm her down, but the daughter reminded her mom that she always taught her children to believe every word of the Bible. She arose from bed, put on her clothes, and shouted throughout the house. She was completely healed!

What happened here? She treated the Word of God as if it was actually *true*! So we see that real faith is taking God at His Word and stepping out upon His promises with all confidence and sincerity, without a doubt or fear!

You can exercise your faith in the same way today and receive your healing!

Day 18

Faith for Healing

Healing is your present possession because Jesus paid the price for it and gave it to you. However, it can only be a reality in your life if you use your faith for it. This is why we emphasize the subject of faith repeatedly.

Hebrews 11:6 says,

> **But without faith it is impossible to please Him, for he who comes to God must believe that He is, and that He is a rewarder of those who diligently seek Him.**

The reason it's impossible to please God without faith is because everything we receive from God requires our faith. And God wants us to receive what He has provided for us. The Bible teaches us that God is love. Love gives, and love wants the gifts to be received!

Now if God requires that we have faith to please Him, and if it were impossible for us to acquire it, we would have a right to challenge His justice. However, since He has given us the ability to obtain faith, then the responsibility rests with us to get it. Thankfully, He has told us how to obtain faith.

> **But what does it say? "The word is near you, in your mouth and in your heart" (that is, the word of faith which we preach): that if you confess with your mouth the Lord Jesus and believe in your heart that God has raised Him from the dead, you will be saved. For with the heart one believes unto righteousness, and with the mouth confession is made unto salvation. (Rom. 10:8-10)**

> **For "whoever calls on the name of the LORD shall be saved." How then shall they call on Him in whom they have not believed? And how shall they believe in Him of whom they have not *heard*? And how shall they hear without a preacher? (Rom. 10:13-14)**

> **So then faith comes by hearing, and hearing by the word of God. (Rom. 10:17)**

These verses give us instructions on how to receive salvation and healing. We see a very important truth here: People are saved and healed by *faith*. We also see that faith is obtained by hearing. Let's look at a few examples.

> **And they were preaching the gospel there. And in Lystra a certain man without strength in his feet was sitting, a cripple from his mother's womb, who had never walked. This man heard**

> **Paul speaking. Paul, observing him intently and seeing that he had faith to be healed, said with a loud voice, "Stand up straight on your feet!" And he leaped and walked. (Acts 14:7-10)**

If you look carefully at this passage, Paul did *not* heal that man. The scriptures say that the man himself had faith to be healed.

1. **He heard Paul preach.**
2. **He had faith to be healed.**
3. **He leaped and walked—he acted on his faith.**

Where did the man get the faith to be healed? By hearing Paul speak. What did Paul speak? He preached the Gospel. Therefore, Paul must have preached a Gospel that included salvation *and* healing!

Paul said this in Romans 1:16:

> **For I am not ashamed of the gospel of Christ, for it is the power of God to salvation for everyone who believes, for the Jew first and also for the Greek.**

The Greek and Hebrew words for *salvation* include the ideas of deliverance, safety, preservation, healing, and soundness. The Gospel is the power of God unto healing and soundness. Paul preached the *full* Gospel, not just part of it!

Here's another great passage:

> **Then Philip went down to the city of Samaria and preached Christ to them. And the multitudes with one accord heeded the things spoken by Philip, hearing and seeing the miracles which he did. For unclean spirits, crying with a loud voice, came out of many who were possessed; and many who were paralyzed and lame were healed. And there was great joy in that city. (Acts 8:5-8)**

These miracles took place as a result of Philip preaching Christ. The New Testament teaches that Christ is the *Savior* and the *Healer*. If there is no Gospel of healing today, then there is no Gospel of salvation. They are inseparable. They are a package deal.

There will always be those who will tell you that healing has been done away with. But can you ever remember hearing that *faith* has been done away with? No, you haven't and you never will! And as long as faith has not been done away with, you can still receive all of God's promises—including healing!

It's too late to tell me healing is not for today. I've been receiving healing for myself and my family for over four decades. I've been blessed to never have received a serious diagnosis, but I have had minor things come up as I've aged. For example, I once was diagnosed with high cholesterol and an elevated TSH level. I did not take any medication for these. I used my faith to change those levels back to normal.

I talked to my body *every* day and commanded my cholesterol and TSH levels to be normal, and both levels returned to normal by my next blood test.

How could I confidently do this? Because faith came when I heard God's word about healing. Then I released my faith by agreeing with God and saying what He says about it. By agreeing and speaking, I acted upon my faith. God is not a respecter of persons. What He did for me He will do for you! Meditate on the Word of God and release your faith by speaking His Word daily.

Day 19

All Things Are Possible

In the book of Mark, we see a story of a man who asked Jesus to help his son. The man's son was mute and was often afflicted with epileptic seizures.

> **"And often he has thrown him both into the fire and into the water to destroy him. But if You can do anything, have compassion on us and help us." Jesus said to him, *"If you can believe, all things are possible to him who believes."* Immediately the father of the child cried out and said with tears, "Lord, I believe; help my unbelief!" (Mark 9:22-24, emphasis mine)**

This man was desperate. I'm sure we all have been in situations where we felt desperate. He begged Jesus for help. He didn't have a full understanding of how healing and deliverance worked. So he said, "*If* you can do anything..." Jesus quickly settled this issue of "*if*."

He basically responded by saying, *"It's not a question of what I can do. The question is, what can you believe? If you can believe, all things are possible for you. It's not up to Me, it's up to you. I don't decide if your son gets healed. You do! I have the ability, but it's up to you whether or not My power is released."*

So often we cry out, "Oh God, do something!" But God always says, "You believe, then I'll move!" It's human nature to want to put all the responsibility on someone else. However, this is not the way God operates. All throughout the scriptures, God put the ball back into the court of the individual who had a need.

Actually, God gave us His Word *and* His faith. He will do anything He has promised if we will simply believe Him. In order to believe God's Word, we must hear it. Then, if we will use the faith He gives us through His Word, He will move for us and supply the need. God really gave us the easy part of the covenant: only *believe*!

Jesus spent a good deal of His time on earth teaching people the Word and will of God so that they could have something to believe. After hearing, they had to act on their faith in that Word. The Bible says that Jesus is the same yesterday, today, and forever. Therefore, by your faith, all things are possible to you today.

When this man came to Jesus for his son's healing, he didn't get discouraged by Jesus' words. He responded by saying, "All right Lord, I believe. Help my unbelief." What does that mean? He was saying, "I believe in my heart, but my head is giving me trouble." Doubts were trying to overtake his mind.

Have you ever faced a situation like that? You know in your heart that what God says is true, but your head is giving you every reason why it isn't working or it can't work. To deal with our head, we must become skillful in looking to the Word, not at the problem or the diagnosis.

Second Corinthians 4:18 says,

> **While we do not look at the things which are seen, but at the things which are not seen. For the things which are seen are temporary, but the things which are not seen are eternal.**

We see the problem is there, but we refuse to be troubled by it. We are to look at God's unseen Word which produces victory every time!

Here's another great scripture:

> **For what if some did not believe? Will their unbelief make the faithfulness of God without effect? Certainly not! Indeed, let God be true but every man a liar. (Rom. 3:3-4)**

This means that we have to let God be true in our lives. God is not a dictator. He always gives us a choice.

First Peter 2:24 says, "By His stripes you were healed." Many would respond by saying, "I know that's what the Bible says, but I don't feel well." They have chosen to let the symptoms be truth and God a liar. You may know God's

Word is true for all people, but Paul said in Romans that you have to choose what is truth in *your* own life. Are you going to believe symptoms and circumstances, or are you going to believe God's Word?

We must always remember that "all things are possible to him that believes" (Mark 9:23). Let's choose to believe God today and receive healing!

Day 20

The Evidence of Your Healing

There are certain established spiritual laws that cause God's power to flow into a person. Spiritual laws are as predictable as natural laws. One very important spiritual law that accesses the power of healing is the law of *faith.* Unless someone releases his faith for healing, healing power will not flow.

What exactly is Bible faith? The biblical definition is found in Hebrews chapter 11, verse 1.

> **Now faith is the substance of things hoped for, the evidence of things not seen.**

Moffatt's translation says:

> **Now faith means that we are confident of what we hope for, *convinced of what we do not see.***

Everyone alive has a natural human faith. Human faith believes in natural facts, like the ability of a chair to hold you up when you sit in it. But this scripture is talking about a supernatural faith. Supernatural faith believes with the heart rather than believing what the physical senses may tell us. Faith will take things that seem unrealistic and bring them into the realm of reality.

This scripture says that faith is the evidence of things *not* seen. You may have sickness or pain in your body, but faith says, "By His stripes I am healed!" Faith will always say about itself everything that the Word of God says. Faith in God is simply faith in His Word.

A dear man of God who greatly impacted my life had a great testimony along these lines. He had been bedfast for sixteen months with an incurable disease as a teenager. Doctors told him he would die, but he stood on God's Word and received a miraculous healing.

He only weighed about ninety pounds when he was first healed, although he stood over six feet tall. Within only a few months, he looked for a job. These were depression days, and jobs were hard to find. He was eventually hired to pull up two-year-old peach trees from the roots. Each day the number of workers was fewer and fewer, and each day someone would say to him, "I didn't think you'd make it today."

His response would always be, "If it weren't for the Lord I wouldn't be here. The Lord is the strength of my life." He said if he had gone by his feelings, he wouldn't have gotten out of bed. Instead, he continually quoted, "The LORD is the strength of my life" (Ps. 27:1).

Here is an interesting point: He said he never received any strength until he started pulling up that first tree. But once he began to put his hands to the trunk of the tree, an anointing would flow over him like honey, and he would work in that supernatural strength all day long. He also ended up being the last person on that job!

Many people want to receive first and only then believe they've got their healing. But it doesn't work that way. You must believe first, and then you will receive. This is called supernatural faith, not head faith.

Jesus explained supernatural faith so well in Mark chapter 11:

> **So Jesus answered and said to them, "Have faith in God. For assuredly, I say to you, whoever says to this mountain, 'Be removed and be cast into the sea,' and does not doubt in his heart, but believes that those things he says will be done, he will have whatever he says. Therefore I say to you, whatever things you ask when you pray, believe that you receive them, and you will have them." (Mark 11:22-24)**

Here is the difference between supernatural faith and mentally agreeing with God's Word:

Mental agreement says, "I know God's Word is true. I know the Word says I'm healed. But for some reason, it's not working for me."

Supernatural faith (real faith in God's Word) **says,** "God cannot lie. Because God's Word is true, I have it now, regardless of what I feel or see."

Many people have said, "But the thing I've been praying about hasn't come to pass yet." If you could feel or see it, you wouldn't need faith for it anymore. You have to take the step of believing *before* you will see it come to pass. Notice Mark 11:24 says that the receiving comes after the believing. Jesus simply said, "You've got to believe you have it before you can receive it" (paraphrased).

I never have received healing without first believing I have it. My body may be shouting at me that I don't have it! However, when I firmly stand on the Word of God, and continue to say what God says, results always come *after* I believe.

If we are going to complain about our symptoms, waiting until they are gone before we believe we are healed, we will never see healing manifest in our bodies.

Remember that faith is the evidence of things *not* seen!

Day 21

See Yourself Healed

Faith always believes we have our answer from God *now*. Faith does not *hope* we will see the answer. The eyes of faith see the answer as having already happened! How is this possible? Through placing our attention on the right things.

Proverbs 4:20-22 says,

> **My son, give attention to my words;**
> **Incline your ear to my sayings.**
> **Do not let them depart from your eyes;**
> **Keep them in the midst of your heart;**
> **For they are life to those who find them,**
> **And health to all their flesh.**

Notice this passage says to not let God's words depart from your eyes. Many people fail because they see themselves as failing; their eyes are on failing, not on God's Word. Some who are sick see themselves as dying.

Matthew 8:17 says,

> **He Himself took our infirmities**
> **And bore our sicknesses.**

If that Word does not depart from before our eyes, we will eventually see ourselves well. However, if we stop meditating upon the healing promises of God, we will begin to see ourselves as sick and trying to obtain healing. We must keep God's Word in the midst of our heart in order for health to become a reality in our life.

Look again at Proverbs 4:20-22:

> **"My Words... are life to those who find them, and health to all their flesh."**

The Hebrew word translated *health* here is also the word for *medicine*. God's words are medicine to all our flesh. Just like natural medicine must be taken as prescribed, God's medicine must be taken according to His directions. And one of the instructions is to not let them depart from your eyes. We are to continue to meditate upon the Word of God until we see ourselves with the promise.

If you continue to envision everything getting worse, all the praying in the world won't do you a bit of good. Focusing on the wrong thing will destroy the effects of prayer. Instead, constantly confess that you are already healed because the Word of God says you are. Picture yourself as having already received your healing. That's when you will get results.

> **While we do not look at the things which are seen, but at the things which are not seen. For the things which are seen are temporary, but the things which are not seen are eternal. (2 Cor. 4:18)**

Faith will always contradict negative circumstances. For example, 1 Peter 2:24 says, "By whose stripes, you were healed."

Are we saying, "I am healed"? This is what we should be declaring. Yet so many say, "I don't feel well. I'm sick. I'm dying." That is because they are looking at things that are seen instead of looking at what the Word of God says.

If our eyes are on what the Lord promises, "By whose stripes you were healed," then we can boldly declare, "I *am* healed!" Let's quit saying the wrong things and start saying the right things. Wrong seeing, wrong thinking, wrong believing, and wrong talking will defeat us. The devil cannot defeat us because Jesus has already defeated the devil for us. But we can defeat ourselves by *seeing* and *saying* the wrong things.

We must keep the Word before our eyes so we can believe and say the right things. Faith not only sees the answer, but it will always say the answer. Saying it more will actually cause us to see it more! Start seeing yourself healed today, and you will soon enjoy the reality of it!

Day 22

Healing Is Not a Feeling

A man of faith once said, "I can't understand God by feelings. I can't understand the Lord Jesus Christ by feelings. I can only understand God and Jesus by what the Word says about them."

Too many people try to get to know God by their feelings. When they feel good, they think God heard their prayers. When they don't feel good, they conclude that He has not heard them. Their faith is based on their feelings when it should be based on the Word of God.

This is the problem Thomas had. He was not with the other disciples when Jesus appeared to them the first time. Because he didn't see Jesus, he refused to believe what all the others told him. Thomas said, "Unless I see Him and touch Him for myself, I will not believe."

Eight days later, Jesus appeared to them again. This time Thomas was present. He refused to believe unless he could see with his own eyes and feel Jesus' wounds with his own hands.

> **Then He said to Thomas, "Reach your finger here, and look at My hands; and reach your hand here, and put it into My side. Do not be unbelieving, but believing." (John 20:27)**

Many Christians are like Thomas. They refuse to believe they are healed because they don't feel any different after they pray and they don't see the evidence. Needing to feel a change or see evidence is not Bible faith. For it is by faith —not by sight or evidence—that we receive. So if we require a feeling or evidence before we believe, healing won't manifest in our bodies.

Real faith in God is based upon the Word of God. Real faith says, "If God's Word says it is true, then it is. If God's Word says I'm healed, then I am healed, because His Word cannot lie." God's Word is always true, regardless of our feelings or circumstances.

When it comes to the physical realm, we have to walk by sight. But when it comes to spiritual things, we don't walk by sight, we walk by faith. "*For we walk by faith, not by sight*" (2 Cor. 5:7).

God's healing takes place in the spirit realm. If medical science heals, it heals through the physical body. Christian Science teaches that healing comes through the mind. But when God heals, He heals through the spirit of man. Although we cannot see into the spirit realm with our natural eyes, it is still very real. That's where faith comes into play.

Healing is like the New Birth. The New Birth is the rebirth of the human spirit. It does not change the physical in any way, so it is not seen with the natural eyes. However, over time it should become obvious that there has been a change.

In the same way, healing from God begins in the spirit of man. To receive physical healing, we must believe with our spirits. Only then will we feel or see the difference. The Bible addresses our spirits first and foremost; healing in our bodies always starts in the spirit.

Here is a formula for faith that will work for you:

1. **Find one or two healing scriptures that are meaningful to you.** Personalize them by inserting your name.

2. **Meditate upon them until you know in your heart you believe them.**

3. **Refuse to consider contradictory circumstances or what your physical senses may tell you.** Don't allow your feelings or senses to talk you out of your healing.

4. **Continually praise God that you are healed!**

Day 23

Authority Over Sickness

There is a word that is almost lost to our society today: *redemption*. Redemption is the act of saving or being saved from sin and evil. Another definition is the action of regaining possession of something in exchange for payment, or of clearing a debt.

What did God regain for you and me?
Forgiveness and healing!

What was exchanged for payment?
The precious blood of Jesus.

Now why is this so important for you to understand? Because until you really understand the reality of your redemption in Christ, you will not be able to live in health. The blood of Jesus has redeemed you from the authority of Satan! By receiving Jesus as your Lord, you were translated out of the authority of Satan and into the Kingdom of God.

Colossians 1:13-14 says,

> **He has delivered us from the power of darkness and conveyed us into the kingdom of the Son of His love, in whom we have redemption through His blood, the forgiveness of sins.**

The word *power* in verse thirteen actually means *authority.*

Notice two things:

1. **We *have been* delivered from Satan's authority —we're not *going* to be someday in the future.**
2. **The price of redemption was the blood of Jesus.**

Here's another scripture in connection with this:

> **And they overcame him by the blood of the Lamb and by the word of their testimony. (Rev. 12:11)**

The American Standard Version says it this way:

> **Because of the blood of the Lamb, and because of the word of their testimony.**

The blood of Jesus is the basis for our victory! He paid the price. Legally, we are free from all sickness, disease, and pain. Now that we know we are free from these, we must enforce our legal standing by adding our confession to it. What are we saying about our redemption? We have to stand our ground against the enemy by speaking with the authority God gave us to declare our redemption.

Because Satan is the god of this world, he will try to exercise authority over us, even though he has been stripped of it. But he never has to win! Why? Because we have been delivered by the blood of the Lamb from all the power of darkness. In every test of sickness, disease, or any other evil, we can overcome. How? Through our agreement. If we don't agree with God, we will not enjoy His provision. You agree by saying what He has said about the situation. The word of our testimony should always be, "I am healed, I am redeemed by the blood of the Lamb." That is called taking authority.

Think about this: We belong to the body of Christ. Christ is the head of that body, and He rules over His body. Satan has no right to rule over Christ, therefore he has no right to rule over Christ's body.

Some people accept defeat in life because they don't fully understand these truths. They often believe that it is God's will for them to be sick and defeated. But why would God want someone that belongs to Him to be defeated in any way?

First Corinthians 6:19-20 says,

> **Or do you not know that your body is the temple of the Holy Spirit who is in you, whom you have from God, and you are not your own? For you were bought at a price; therefore glorify God in your body and in your spirit, which are God's.**

This passage shows us that not only our spirit, but also our body was bought with a price. Therefore, we are to glorify God in our body and in our spirit, which now belong to God. He paid for us—He owns us—and therefore He is glorified by our healed bodies.

Could God get any glory out of the body, the temple of the Holy Spirit, if it is deformed with sickness? We must understand that our healed bodies reflect God's glory. Knowing this will embolden us to take a firm stand against the devil when he attacks our bodies. Our authority over Satan, sin, and sickness is part of our inheritance in Christ.

We have dominion over the devil because of the blood of the Lamb, and because of the word of our testimony. We have already overcome Satan. We can glorify God in our spirits and our bodies *now*. But we must believe the authority that is ours through the blood of Jesus, and we must confess that it has healed us of every sickness and disease.

Day 24

A Healing Tongue

One of the most important things to understand about divine healing is that you will never receive it without getting in agreement with God. Receiving divine healing requires your cooperation in two main areas. You must believe God's Word, and you must speak God's Word on a continual basis.

You will never change your physical condition without believing right and speaking right. Believing accurately is only possible if you guard your thought life and think accurately first. We would all like to pride ourselves in believing that our thoughts are always right. However, the first step to cooperating with God is acknowledging that your thoughts may not agree with God's. Then, you can begin obtaining God's thoughts.

Isaiah 55:8-9 says,

> **"For My thoughts are not your thoughts,**
> **Nor are your ways My ways," says the Lord.**
> **"For as the heavens are higher than the earth,**
> **So are My ways higher than your ways,**
> **And My thoughts than your thoughts."**

If you want to know exactly what you've been thinking and believing, start paying attention to what you regularly *say*. Jesus said, "For out of the abundance of the heart the mouth speaks" (Matt. 12:34).

Many do not realize that their words determine the course of their life. James 3:2 tells us, "For we all stumble in many things. If anyone does not stumble in word, he is a perfect man, able also to bridle the whole body." If you can control what you say, you can control the outcome of your health. If you continually talk about sickness and pain, you will continue to have sickness and pain. However, if you continually say what God says about your body, healing will begin to manifest in your body.

Here are a few more scriptures that reveal the power of the tongue:

> **The tongue can bring death or life;**
> **those who love to talk will reap the consequences. (Prov. 18:21 NLT)**
>
> **A gentle tongue [with its healing power] is a tree of life. (Prov. 15:4 AMPC)**

Remember that the tree of life was in the garden of Eden, and if Adam and Eve would have eaten of it first, they would have lived on earth forever in health and peace.

Here's something else worth noting about words. When God wants something to come to pass, He speaks it first. We see the first example of this in the book of Genesis.

Then God said, "Let there be light"; and there was light. (Gen. 1:3)

Because we have been created in God's likeness, we also have the ability to speak things into existence. Jesus taught us this truth in Mark 11:23.

"For assuredly, I say to you, whoever says to this mountain, 'Be removed and be cast into the sea,' and does not doubt in his heart, but believes that those things he says will be done, he will have whatever he says."

Since we will have what we believe and say, we should be watchful over our hearts and our words. We should be agreeing with God by saying what He says about any area of our lives. Let's look again at what God says about our health.

"He Himself took our infirmities
And bore our sicknesses." (Matt. 8:17-18)

By whose stripes you were healed. (1 Pet. 2:24)

Through the process of meditation, you will get to the place where you believe this in your heart and confess it with your mouth, and that is exactly what you will have.

There is a spiritual law that few realize: Our confessions rule us. Sooner or later, everyone will have what they confess in life. All of us have two choices on a daily basis. We can talk about what the devil is doing, or we can talk about what God has done and what we have in Christ.

The more we talk about the symptoms in our bodies, the more we glorify what the devil is doing, and the more we have sickness and disease. The more we talk about the Word of God, the more we glorify God, and the more we will have health and healing in our bodies. Our faith will actually keep pace with our confession. Another way to say this is that faith never rises above its confession.

Nothing will drain you of faith faster than speaking against God's Word. If you expect to receive the healing that God has provided, you must master your tongue.

The solution for overcoming a negative confession is keeping your heart filled with the Word of God in abundance. It will then be natural for you to say what God says about your health. Remember, your tongue can minister healing power to your body and direct your life into divine health.

Day 25

Peace Is Our Inheritance

Jesus not only paid the price for the complete and total healing of our bodies. He also paid the price for the peace of our minds. If our minds are not peaceful, it will eventually lead to sickness in our bodies. Medical science tells us that about 80% of all illness stems from poor mental health. Many have struggled with anxiety and depression for a long time and wonder if there is any hope for them. I want you to know that there absolutely is hope to overcome mental oppression.

Isaiah 53:5 from the Amplified Classic translation says,

> **But He was wounded for our transgressions, He was bruised for our guilt and iniquities; the chastisement [needful to obtain] peace and well-being for us was upon Him, and with the stripes [that wounded] Him we are healed and made whole.**

Notice that Jesus was chastised—it was necessary to obtain peace and well-being for us. In the same way that

Jesus paid the price for our sins and our diseases, He paid the price for anxiety and depression! And the same way that we receive forgiveness and healing, we also receive our peace and well-being. *By faith!*

Peace in life is everything! Jesus knows this to be true. He said in John 14:27,

> **Peace I leave with you, My peace I give to you; not as the world gives do I give to you. Let not your heart be troubled, neither let it be afraid.**

In the Amplified Classic translation it says,

> **Peace I leave with you, My [own] peace I now give and bequeath to you.**

According to Merriam-Webster's dictionary, to *bequeath* is "to give or leave by will; to hand down". Jesus willed to you an inheritance of His very own peace!

It's important to note that Jesus talked about two types of peace in the passage we read.

1. **The peace that Jesus gives.**
2. **The peace that the world gives.**

The peace the world offers is a feeling of security based on favorable circumstances. As long as everything is going our way—we have enough money, we are healthy, or there are no conflicts in our lives—we feel at peace. The problem with this peace is that it is fragile and fleeting. As soon as a circumstance changes for the worse, the peace goes away and anxiety and worry rush in to fill the void. The world doesn't have any lasting peace to offer us. Satan only offers an illusion of peace that will always leave us with disappointment.

If we want true, lasting peace, we won't find it in this world. Apart from Jesus, Satan will steal, kill, and destroy anything good in our lives. But thank God, there is another kind of peace available to us when we are born again—the peace Jesus offers. His peace will keep us calm and content regardless of the circumstances.

You may be wondering, "If I have the peace of God, why do I feel so troubled?" The reason so many believers are not experiencing God's peace is because the enemy has manipulated their emotions. The fact is, you will feel many different emotions throughout your lifetime, and your feelings are attached to your thoughts.

Satan's primary target is your mind. His strategy is to suggest a troubling thought to you and accompany that thought with a feeling, which makes it seem real.

For example, here's one he has tried with all of us. He will interject a thought into your mind that says, "I'm worthless." Along with that thought, he will attach a sinking feeling of condemnation and guilt. He will almost always bring up a past failure.

If you don't know who you are in Christ, you will surrender your peace. Here is a very important point: It is vital for us to know God's Word so we can quickly recognize the lies of the devil and cast them down.

The way we really get to know the Word of God is by renewing our minds to think God's thoughts.

Romans 12:2 says,

> **And do not be conformed to this world, but be transformed by the renewing of your mind, that you may prove what is that good and acceptable and perfect will of God.**

Here is how it's done:

1. **Find scriptures that pertain to whatever you are tempted to be fearful about.**
2. **Meditate upon those scriptures day and night.**
3. **When thoughts come to your mind that contradict God's Word, speak the Word only, not the negative thoughts.**

Your renewed mind will recognize and reject ungodly and fearful thoughts, like the thought of worthlessness we talked about earlier. It will also reject thoughts of living with disease the rest of your life, or thoughts of premature death. Rejecting unscriptural thoughts is *faith* in action. And faith in God's Word keeps us in the perfect peace that we inherited from Jesus our Lord.

For further teaching on peace, please reference my book *Untroubled: Conquering Anxiety, Fear, and Depression.*

Day 26

Don't Call It Like You See It

Have you ever heard someone say about situations, "I just call things like I see them"? Or have you seen the slogan, "Seeing is Believing"? I'm sure these people take pride in what they think is honesty.

However, these phrases actually contradict the Word of God. If you keep saying what you see, you will keep on having what you see. If what you see is not what you want, you will have to change what you are saying. I'll prove this to you from the scriptures.

Let's first look at what Jesus said about this:

> **So Jesus answered and said to them, "Have faith in God. For assuredly, I say to you, whoever says to this mountain, 'Be removed and be cast into the sea' and does not doubt in his heart, but believes that those things he *says* will be done, he will have whatever he *says*." (Mark 11:22-23, emphasis mine)**

Jesus is showing us that our words matter. He is also showing us how the faith of God operates, and then tells us to do the same thing. A more literal translation of "Have faith in God" is "Have the faith *of* God"! We see how the faith of God operates in creation in Genesis.

> **And God said, Let there be light: and there was light. (Gen. 1:3 KJV)**
>
> **And God said, Let the waters under the heaven be gathered together unto one place, and let the dry land appear: and it was so. (Gen. 1:9 KJV)**
>
> **And God said, Let the earth bring forth grass, the herb yielding seed, and the fruit tree yielding fruit after his kind, whose seed is in itself, upon the earth: and it was so. (Gen. 1:11 KJV)**

Everything that God created was done by His faith. Notice He *said* it and it was so. We saw in Mark 11:23 that when we say something and do not doubt in our heart, but believe, we will have whatever *we* say! Faith believes with the heart and speaks with the mouth! Faith says the desired outcome before ever seeing it.

We see this very principle in the life of Abraham.

> **As it is written, I have made you the father of many nations. [He was appointed our father] in the sight of God in Whom he believed, Who gives life to the dead and speaks of the nonexistent things that [He has foretold and promised] as if they [already] existed. (Rom. 4:17 AMPC)**

The King James version says,

> **Even God, Who quickeneth the dead, and calleth those things that be not as though they were.**

Many have argued, "That's God. He can do that." But we know that Abraham did the same thing that God did. He had a struggle for a while. For around 24 years, he and Sarah still did not have the promised child. So God came along and helped his faith. God changed his name. He was called Abram, but then God changed his name to Abraham.

Abraham means "the father of a multitude." Going forward, every time someone addressed him, they called him "father of a multitude." Every time he introduced himself, he said out of his own mouth, "I'm the father of a multitude."

> **No unbelief or distrust made him waver (doubtingly question) concerning the promise of God, but he grew strong and was empowered by faith as he gave praise and glory to God. (Rom. 4:20 AMPC)**

Notice that Abraham grew strong and was empowered by faith as he gave praise and glory to God. One way that we give glory to God is to agree with Him. The way we agree is to say the same thing that God says about us.

Hebrews 4:14 says,

> **Seeing then that we have a great High Priest who has passed through the heavens, Jesus the Son of God, let us hold fast our confession.**

The Greek translation for the last part of that verse is, "Let us hold fast to saying the same things." We are to hold fast to saying the same things that God is saying about us and our situations.

First Peter 2:24 says, "By whose stripes you *were* healed." We are to hold fast to saying we *were* healed, regardless of our symptoms.

This is what Abraham did.

> **He did not weaken in faith when he considered the [utter] impotence of his own body, which was as good as dead because he was about a hundred years old, or [when he considered] the barrenness of Sarah's [deadened] womb. (Rom. 4:19 AMPC)**

Abraham and Sarah had symptoms of barrenness. If Sarah was 16 when she married Abraham, which would not have been uncommon in that day, they would have tried for nearly seventy-five years to get pregnant. Think about that the next time you believe your situation is hopeless!

But because Abraham finally began to say what God said, he began to call those things that did not exist in the natural as though they already did—he got to the place where he no longer considered the natural condition of their bodies.

And then he became fully convinced in his heart:

> **And being fully convinced that what He had promised He was also able to perform. (Rom. 4:21)**

Just as Abraham did, we too will become fully convinced that we are healed if we will agree with God and say what God says continually. Don't say it like you see it in the natural. Say what God says, and you will have your healing!

Day 27

The Fight of Faith

Many people are not living in health or receiving divine healing when they need it. One reason is because authority must be exercised over disease. We live in a fallen world that is governed by Satan, who is called "the god of this world" (2 Cor. 4:4). Satan hates what God loves most, and therefore he hates humanity with a passion. He seeks to disrupt the will of God in every area.

> **The thief does not come except to steal, and to kill, and to destroy. I have come that they may have life, and that they may have it more abundantly. (John 10:10)**

Even though Satan has legally been defeated by Jesus, he will try to operate on this earth illegally. How is this possible? It is illegal to murder, and yet renegades are murdering people daily worldwide. In order to stop illegal activity, somebody has to enforce the laws. This is the same way the Kingdom of God operates on the earth. God needs someone with authority to enforce Satan's defeat. If believers don't enforce Satan's defeat, he will continue to illegally steal, kill, and destroy.

The only people who are authorized in the earth to withstand Satan are those who have accepted Jesus as their Lord and Savior. This is because it takes the power of the Holy Spirit to resist the devil, and only those who are born again have the Holy Spirit living in them.

When it comes to *your* health, *you* are the one authorized to enforce Satan's defeat. You must learn to stand your ground and expel sickness, or the devil will illegally try to put things on you that don't belong to you.

> **So be subject to God. Resist the devil [stand firm against him], and he will flee from you. (James 4:7 AMPC)**

We have to understand that resisting the devil requires faith. And the Bible makes it clear that faith is not passive. It has a *fight* to it!

> **Fight the good fight of faith. (1 Tim. 6:12)**

The only fight the Christian is called to fight in this life is the faith fight! If we are in any other kind of fight, we are in the wrong fight. Some have said, "I'm going to fight the devil," or "I'm fighting this sickness or disease." Nobody has to fight the devil or sickness! Why? Because Jesus already defeated them. We need to get out of the wrong fight and get into the right one.

You may ask, "If we are not fighting the devil, then what are we fighting?" We are fighting *doubt* and *unbelief*. We are fighting to stay in faith about our healing, or about anything else the Word of God promises us.

God's Word always tells the truth! God's Word says, "By whose stripes you were healed." However, our bodies and the devil will try to sway us into doubt and unbelief about the truth that we *were* healed. This is where the faith fight begins. We must learn to stand our ground in the face of Satan's believable lies.

How do we fight the good fight of faith for healing? Here are four simple steps:

1. **Meditate upon the Word of God daily.**

   This Book of the Law shall not depart from your mouth, but you shall meditate in it day and night, that you may observe to do according to all that is written in it. For then you will make your way prosperous, and then you will have good success. (Josh. 1:8)

   Find one or two healing scriptures that stir your spirit and meditate upon them daily. Meditate means to ponder and mutter. Say those scriptures out loud throughout the day and put yourself into those verses.

2. **Act like the Word of God is true.**

   According to Joshua 1:8 the purpose of meditation is to get us to the place where we do what the Word says. If you can't move a limb, attempt to move it. If you have the flu and are lying in bed, get out of bed. Act as far as you can with your faith.

One of the greatest acts of faith is simply agreeing with God by saying only what He says about your situation. Continue to confess that you are already healed according to 1 Peter 2:24, regardless of what you feel in your body.

3. **Don't consider your body more than what God says.**

   We must give a certain amount of attention to symptoms in order to evaluate how to address them. However, worrying about our symptoms will never lead to healing. We must stay focused on what God says about it.

4. **Never quit!**

   And let us not grow weary while doing good, for in due season we shall reap if we do not lose heart. (Gal. 6:9)

   Refuse to be moved from your stand of faith. If you keep your spirit fortified with the Word of God, you will have the strength to stand for as long as needed.

We see now why many are not walking in divine health. Many have not fought the good fight of faith. But I want to encourage you to be one who does engage in the faith fight! The fight of faith is called the *good* fight because real faith in God's Word always wins.

Day 28

The Battle for Healing Is the Lord's, But the Victory Is Yours

We must learn to let the Lord fight our battles. The battle is the Lord's, and what's more, He already won it! This means the victory is ours now! We don't need to defeat the devil, because he is already defeated.

> **And having spoiled principalities and powers, he made a shew of them openly, triumphing over them in it. (Col. 2:15 KJV)**
>
> **For the battle is the LORD's. (1 Sam. 17:47)**

Many don't understand that the battle's already been won by God. They mistakenly think they must win it by praying long and hard enough. Prayer is important, but it's never our struggling in prayer that earns health and healing from God. Healing is not a reward for good works. Healing is the property of every believer. The main work of the believer is the work of believing—the work of faith.

> **Then they said to Him, "What shall we do, that we may work the works of God?"**
>
> **Jesus answered and said to them, "This is the work of God, that you *believe* in Him whom He sent." (John 6:28-29)**

Since the main work of the believer is the work of faith, our minds have become Satan's battleground. He seeks to sway us into doubt and unbelief regarding our victory so that we cannot enjoy it. When we put God's Word to work for us, the Word fights our mental battles for us. It keeps our minds focused on truth rather than symptoms. We have to realize that the place of faith is a place of rest, not struggle.

> **Therefore, since a promise remains of entering His rest, let us fear lest any of you seem to have come short of it. For indeed the gospel was preached to us as well as to them; but the word which they heard did not profit them, not being mixed with faith in those who heard it. For we who have believed do enter that rest. (Heb. 4:1-3)**

Faith for healing can only come through the Word of God. And yet, many who actually hear still do not receive healing. It does not profit them. Why? Because faith must be mixed with the Word we hear in order to put the Word to work for us. How do we mix our faith with the Word? *Our tongue is the mixer.*

It's not enough to just hear God's Word. We must agree with it. If we are not speaking His Word, then we are not agreeing with His Word. I never have been able to receive healing for myself without agreeing with God by speaking His Word.

Some receive a bad diagnosis and become gripped with fear. Fear will often drive a person to pray hard and fast. But fear can also drive a person to speak against the Word of God and instead talk about the diagnosis. They may say things like, "I'm afraid I'm going to die."

You can be praying, but as long as you focus on the diagnosis instead of on the fact that the battle is already won, God cannot perform His Word for you. This is where the work of faith comes in. We work to keep our hearts full of the Word of God, mix it with faith, and speak the Word only. We resist fear by speaking to it and telling it to go.

We don't deny the diagnosis, but we have a more powerful Word from God that will change the diagnosis.

> **"He Himself took our infirmities**
> **And bore our sicknesses." (Matt. 8:17)**

When our firstborn daughter was only five months old, she fell from her day cradle and hit the side of her head with a hard blow. Of course, she began to scream and cry. We laid our hands on her and claimed healing. However, after thirty minutes, she was still crying, and her head had swollen to nearly twice the size. We took her to the emergency room to be examined, but never expected the diagnosis that we received: She had a subdural hematoma, which is bleeding between the brain and the skull, and a depressed fractured skull. She was immediately transferred to a larger, more prominent hospital. They gave the same diagnosis: She would likely have brain damage, or she could die without surgery.

I was a newer believer at this time in my life, but I recognized that I had to guard my heart and mouth with intense watchfulness. We spoke the Word of God only, prayed in the spirit, and worshiped all night long. By the next morning, the tests were repeated and the neurosurgeon gave us the report: There was no trace of bleeding in her brain. It had completely disappeared! He said out of his own mouth that we had received a miracle, and we had the test results to prove it. It was medically impossible for all the bleeding to disappear in one night.

The key here is that we refused to speak anything contrary to the Word of God. Nobody is fully convinced that they are healed when they are speaking against the Word. But if we will mix our faith with a healing scripture by saying it out of our mouths continually, it will surely come to pass.

Being assured of these things causes us to enter a place of rest. Having peace and rest in the midst of a storm is the best way to enjoy the victory that is already yours. The devil will tremble when you enter into faith's rest because he is assured that he's whipped.

Always remember, the battle is the Lord's and the victory is yours!

Day 29

Keep Your Eyes on Jesus

"He Himself took our infirmities and bore our sicknesses."

—Matthew 8:17

Thank God, Jesus bore our sicknesses! From God's perspective, we are legally healed. It is a finished work. Now, if we *are* healed, what do we do when symptoms of disease are raging in our bodies, shouting at us that we are not healed? *We keep our eyes on Jesus!*

The Bible tells us that Jesus and the Word of God are one.

In the beginning was the Word, and the Word was with God, and the Word was God. (John 1:1)

And the Word became flesh and dwelt among us, and we beheld His glory, the glory as of the only begotten of the Father, full of grace and truth (John 1:14)

The way we keep our eyes on Jesus is to keep our eyes on the Word of God. One of the best stories in the Bible to illustrate this is in Matthew.

> **Now in the fourth watch of the night Jesus went to them, walking on the sea. And when the disciples saw Him walking on the sea, they were troubled, saying, "It is a ghost!" And they cried out for fear.**
>
> **But immediately Jesus spoke to them, saying, "Be of good cheer! It is I; do not be afraid."**
>
> **And Peter answered Him and said, "Lord, if it is You, command me to come to You on the water."**
>
> **So He said, "Come." And when Peter had come down out of the boat, he walked on the water to go to Jesus. But when he saw that the wind was boisterous, he was afraid; and beginning to sink he cried out, saying, "Lord, save me!"**
>
> **And immediately Jesus stretched out His hand and caught him, and said to him, "O you of little faith, why did you doubt?" (Matt. 14:25-32)**

Although this is a story about walking on water and not about receiving healing, the same principles apply.

1. **In the natural, it is impossible for a person to walk on water.** It is also impossible for some diseases to be healed medically.

2. **It was only possible to walk on water after Peter knew the will of the Lord.** It is also only possible to receive divine healing when we know the will of the Lord.

How did Peter know the will of God for walking on water? He had the Word of the Lord, "Come." Romans 10:17 says, "Faith comes by hearing, and hearing by the word of God."

Faith came to Peter through that one word, and he stepped out of the boat because of it. How do we know the will of God concerning our healing? It comes from the Word of God, the Bible.

We began by quoting Matthew 8:17, "He Himself took our infirmities, And bore our sicknesses." That is just one verse. A pastor friend of ours did an exhaustive study over several years, searching out every healing scripture in the Bible from 430 translations. He ended up with 454 verses from the Bible on the subject of healing, conclusively proving that healing is the will of God for today. We definitely do not lack for words from God on the subject of healing.

When we hear those words of healing, faith comes. As long as we stay focused on what God says about our healing, we will receive our healing. However, even when we have the Word of the Lord, if we don't stay focused on that Word, the raging storm will pull our attention away from it.

This is what happened to Peter. When he saw that the wind was boisterous, he became fearful. Fear is the opposite of faith. That fear is what caused Peter to lose sight of what Jesus had said and to start sinking. We can see that where our attention goes, our faith goes.

Fighting the good fight of faith is really fighting to keep our attention on the right thing.

> **My son, give attention to my words;**
> **Incline your ear to my sayings.**
> **Do not let them depart from your eyes;**
> **Keep them in the midst of your heart;**
> **For they are life to those who find them,**
> **And health to all their flesh. (Prov. 4:20-23)**

These verses tell us we need to hear God's Word, read God's Word, say God's Word, and act on God's Word. When we keep our attention on God's Word, we are keeping our attention on Jesus, and it becomes medicine to all our flesh. However, we also need to keep our eyes off the raging symptoms and the negative reports. Sometimes this can be challenging. But diligently fixing our eyes on the Word and Jesus actually makes it easier to keep our attention off of the symptoms.

Once we've meditated upon healing scriptures for a period of time, we are ready to believe we receive our healing. Then, one of the best things we can do to keep our attention on the Lord is to lift our hands and worship Him. Thank Him for being such a wonderful Healer.

We worship Him because we are *already* healed, not going to be.

Since it's impossible to think two thoughts at the same time, when we worship the Lord out loud, we cannot be focused on our symptoms. If we continue to look to Jesus, our faith will hold us up, and we will find that our symptoms will disappear.

Day 30

Divine Healing Is Easy

Ah, Lord God! Behold, You have made the heavens and the earth by Your great power and outstretched arm. There is nothing too hard for You.

—Jeremiah 32:17

Divine healing is EASY!

Most people have no difficulty believing that God will forgive them of their sins. But they struggle to believe that a loving God could or would heal them of sickness or disease. With the help of Satan, mankind has made divine healing difficult to receive. But God has always made it easy. One sacrifice, the blood of Jesus and the stripes He bore, redeemed us from every sin and every disease.

We have many types and shadows of this under the Old Covenant.

Bless the Lord, O my soul,
And forget not all His benefits:
Who forgives all your iniquities,
Who heals *all* your diseases. (Ps. 103:2-3)

Notice the word *all* in verse three. That means no sin or disease remains. They have all been forgiven and healed! Every last one, including diseases unknown in Jesus' time.

Verses four and five are so good, I just have to mention them here, too.

> **Who redeems your life from destruction,**
> **Who crowns you with lovingkindness and tender mercies,**
> **Who satisfies your mouth with good things,**
> **So that your youth is renewed like the eagle's.**
> **(Ps. 103:4-5)**

This is the all-inclusive package! These verses show us everything that's included in God's benefits package. We've been redeemed from destruction—that includes cancer and all other destructive diseases. We've been given good and powerful words to speak out of our mouths. The Word of God brings health like a medicine.

Even as we age, we can expect our youth to be renewed. I declare daily that my youth is renewed like the eagle's, and you should too! That's how we stay strong and active in old age.

Let's look at an account of Jesus ministering to a paralytic that validates Psalm 103.

> **"Which is easier, to say to the paralytic, 'Your sins are forgiven you,' or to say, 'Arise, take up your bed and walk'? But that you may know that the Son of Man has power on earth to forgive**

> **sins"—He said to the paralytic, "I say to you, arise, take up your bed, and go to your house." Immediately he arose, took up the bed, and went out in the presence of them all, so that all were amazed and glorified God, saying, "We never saw anything like this!" (Mark 2:9-12)**

Notice the phrase, "Which is *easier*?" Jesus didn't say, "Which is more difficult?" He said, "Which is *easier*?" God thinks that forgiveness and healing are *easy*. People often think that it's hard to receive healing, but that is clearly not God's thought.

> **"For My thoughts are not your thoughts,**
> **Nor are your ways My ways," says the LORD.**
> **"For as the heavens are higher than the earth,**
> **So are My ways higher than your ways,**
> **And My thoughts than your thoughts." (Isa. 55:8-9)**

When it comes to healing, I'm so glad God has higher thoughts than men do! One of His thoughts is: *Forgiveness and healing are both EASY!* Jesus said it was easy to heal a paralytic. There are few things that seem more impossible than a paralytic getting up and walking away completely healed. But remember that Jeremiah said there is nothing too difficult for God!

When we think of something easy, we think of a state of rest. Hebrews 4:3 says, "For we who have believed do enter that rest". When we believe the Word of God, healing becomes easy.

We're going to look at one more witness from the epistles that healing and forgiveness are an easy package deal.

> **Is anyone among you sick? Let him call for the elders of the church, and let them pray over him, anointing him with oil in the name of the Lord. And the prayer of faith will *save* the sick, and the Lord will raise him up. And if he has committed sins, he will be forgiven. (James 5:14-15)**

The word *save* is translated from the Greek word *sozo* which means to heal, preserve, save, do well, and be made whole. The prayer of faith *will* heal the sick. The Lord will raise him up. And if he has sinned, he *will* be forgiven.

This doesn't sound hard to me. This actually sounds *easy*. The next time you're tempted to make healing difficult in your life, remember these words from the Bible. God wants you to live in health so much that He made receiving your healing *easy*!

Day 31

What to Do When Things Get Worse

Many people have said, "I've taken a stand for my healing, but things got worse instead of better!" I want to share with you how to handle a situation like this. The Bible says that there is nothing new under the sun. If your experience is that things got worse after believing, I want you to know you're not alone.

Going all the way back to the children of Israel in Egypt, we see they faced the same dilemma. They had been slaves in Egypt for about 400 years. Slavery was not the will of God for them. So God raised up a deliverer named Moses and sent him back to Egypt.

> **Then Moses and Aaron went and gathered together all the elders of the children of Israel. And Aaron spoke all the words which the LORD had spoken to Moses. Then he did the signs in the sight of the people. So the people *believed*. (Exod. 4:29-31)**

Notice that the people *believed*. Four hundred years is a long time for a negative condition. But they heard good news and they believed. If you've been suffering from a disease for an extended period, you can still believe and receive your healing!

Now, I want you to see that anytime God gives us a good word and we receive it with joy, the devil will be sure to try to hinder that word from coming to pass! He knows that God's word alone will not get the job done. It will always require our *faith* in order for it to come to pass. So Satan seeks to get us into fear, doubt, and unbelief before we see the answer!

After Moses and Aaron visited Pharaoh and gave him the Word of God, do you think Pharaoh was simply delighted to let them go free? Not hardly!

No, here is what happened:

> **So the same day Pharaoh commanded the taskmasters of the people and their officers, saying, "You shall no longer give the people straw to make brick as before. Let them go and gather straw for themselves. And you shall lay on them the quota of bricks which they made before. You shall not reduce it. For they are idle; therefore they cry out, saying, 'Let us go and sacrifice to our God.' Let more work be laid on the men, that they may labor in it, and let them not regard false words." (Exod. 5:6-9)**

So the people complained to Moses, and Moses complained to God.

So Moses returned to the LORD and said, "Lord, why have You brought trouble on this people? Why is it You have sent me? For since I came to Pharaoh to speak in Your name, he has done evil to this people; neither have You delivered Your people at all." (Exod. 5:22-23)

These people did not have any written word of God to build and develop their faith. They had no strong revelation with which to stand their ground. So the Lord continued to give them words of faith and reassurance to see them through. As many of you know, it took some time before Israel was finally released from bondage. Although things got much worse at first, it ultimately came to pass as the Lord had spoken.

Another example in the Bible of things getting worse as a result of standing on the Word of God is in the book of Daniel. King Nebuchadnezzer built a gold image and commanded the people to bow down and worship it every time a certain song was played. Three Jews who were in charge of different provinces refused to bow down to the image. Of course, they had accusers.

Daniel 3:12 says,

"There are certain Jews whom you have set over the affairs of the province of Babylon: Shadrach, Meshach, and Abed-Nego; these men, O king, have not paid due regard to you. They do not serve your gods or worship the gold image which you have set up."

Satan works through people to falsely accuse the saints. He will also speak accusations to our minds. These accusations often have an element of truth to them, which can make it easier for us to feel condemned and can weaken our faith. The devil is always trying to either weaken or remove the saints from a place of victory. The book of Revelation actually describes him as an accuser.

> **Then I heard a loud voice saying in heaven, "Now salvation, and strength, and the kingdom of our God, and the power of His Christ have come, for the accuser of our brethren, who accused them before our God day and night, has been cast down." (Rev. 12:10)**

Back in the book of Daniel, we see the reaction of the king to the accusations:

> **Then Nebuchadnezzar, in rage and fury, gave the command to bring Shadrach, Meshach, and Abed-Nego... "But if you do not worship, you shall be cast immediately into the midst of a burning fiery furnace. And who is the god who will deliver you from my hands?" (Dan. 3:13, 15)**

Here was the response of the three Jews:

> **"If that is the case, our God whom we serve is able to deliver us from the burning fiery furnace, and He will deliver us from your hand, O king." (Dan. 3:17)**

They refused to budge! They refused to give in. They refused to doubt, even in the face of terrible threats.

The devil doesn't like it when we stand up to him! He hates to lose—but so do we! Never give in to the devil!

We know the end of the story: They were not touched by the fire and came out victorious!

Don't be surprised when threats come against your mind as you take a stand against symptoms of disease and pain. The devil will try to turn the heat up to get you to quit believing and throw in the towel. He will say things like, "You know you won't be healed this time." Or "Your faith must not be working because things are getting worse!"

Always remember that Satan is the father of lies. He authored the first lie and has been lying ever since.

So what do we do if things get worse:

1. **Refuse to fear or doubt.** (See 2 Tim. 1:7)

2. **Double up on God's medicine.** (Read our booklet, *What the Bible Says About Healing.*)

3. **Rejoice and praise God continually for the answer.**

4. **Refuse to quit!** Never give up! Never give in to the devil!

If you will put these four steps into practice, before long you will receive the manifestation of your healing!

Prayer to Receive Healing

Dear Heavenly Father,

I make a confession of faith concerning healing. I believe Jesus took my infirmities and bore my sicknesses according to Matthew 8:17 and by His stripes, I *was* healed (1 Pet. 2:24). Therefore, with great confidence and boldness, I say on the authority of that written Word, *I believe I receive my healing, in the Name of Jesus.*

Sickness, disease, and pain, I speak to you in the name of Jesus and command you to leave my body! I am the property of Almighty God, and I give you no place in me. I stand immovable in full assurance that I have health and healing now, in the mighty Name of Jesus. Amen!

Now, continue to praise your Heavenly Father
for His goodness and mercy in your life!

For another great resource on healing,
you can download our booklet,
What the Bible Says About Healing,
at millerministries.org/books

Prayer to Receive Jesus as Lord and Savior

Dear Heavenly Father,

I come to You in the name of Jesus. Your Word says, "The one who comes to Me I will by no means cast out" (John 6:37). So, I know You won't reject me. You will take me in, and I thank You for it.

You said in Your Word, "If you confess with your mouth the Lord Jesus and believe in your heart that God has raised Him from the dead, you will be saved ...For 'whoever calls on the name of the Lord shall be saved'" (Rom. 10:9, 13).

Father, I believe in my heart that Jesus Christ is Your Son and that He died for my sins and was raised from the dead so I can be in right-standing with You. I am calling on the name of Jesus, so I know that You have saved me right now. Thank You, Father.

If you prayed this prayer from your heart, you are now a born-again child of God. Please let us know so we can celebrate with you and send you some free materials to help you grow in your walk with God.

Please email us at hello@millerministries.org or write to: Miller Ministries, PO Box 6404, Aurora, IL 60598

About the Author

Christine Miller was raised in the Catholic faith and attended a Catholic elementary school. As a teenager, she led worship for the guitar masses on Sundays. Although unusually committed to her church at a young age, Christine knew something was missing spiritually and always had a desire to know God better. It was in 1982, while attending college, that she received Jesus as her Lord and Savior. She went on to graduate from Evanston Hospital School of Nursing and later earned a bachelor's in theology from Life Christian University.

For over forty years, Christine has served full-time in ministry as an associate pastor, teacher, and administrator. She has helped her husband, Dr. Jeff Miller, pioneer three churches, including Abundant Life Family Church in Aurora, Illinois, where they currently pastor. She has conducted crusades, held alumni seminars, and preached in conferences and churches both locally and abroad.

The emphasis of her ministry centers on faith and healing. She also operates in the word of knowledge and gifts of healings. In addition to ministering weekly at Abundant Life Family Church, Christine hosts a YouTube program every Friday where she teaches people how to live victoriously.

Christine Miller is ordained by World Harvest Church (Dufresne Ministries) and is a member of Fresh Oil Fellowship Ministerial Association. Many value her mentorship. If you would like to invite Christine to speak at your church or conference, please contact us at MillerMinistries.org.

LIVE FREE FROM ANXIETY AND DEPRESSION

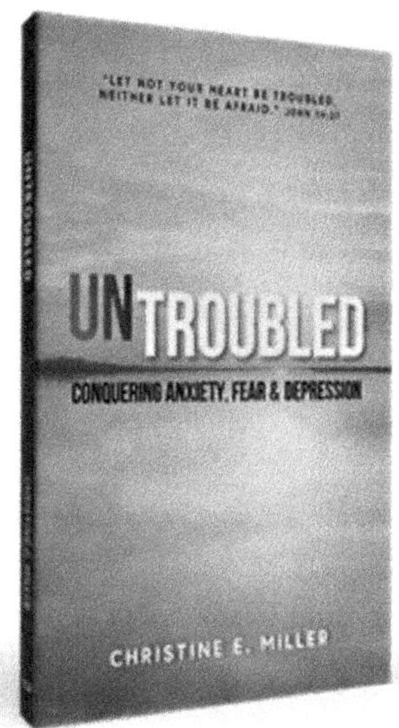

UNTROUBLED
Conquering Anxiety, Fear, and Depression

Christine E. Miller

The world is in a time of great stress and trouble, the likes of which we have never seen. Anxiety, fear, and depression have risen to epidemic levels. Yet in spite of all this, God is able to set us free from fear as we learn to yield to His perfect peace.

In *Untroubled*, Christine Miller shares from the pages of her life, offering time-tested, biblical truth, along with the practical steps needed to navigate your way out of the pit of panic and anxiety and experience freedom from fear in all its forms.

You'll discover...

- What it takes to access your inheritance of peace through Christ
- How to practice thought control
- What a sound mind actually looks like
- The extraordinary value of giving thanks and praise to God
- How God's love expels every trace of fear

Regardless of how challenging life's circumstances may be, they are no match for Jesus! Through the power of His Word and the strength of His Spirit, you can overcome and learn to live in His peace by abiding in Him—your secret place.

Available at **millerministries.org/books**

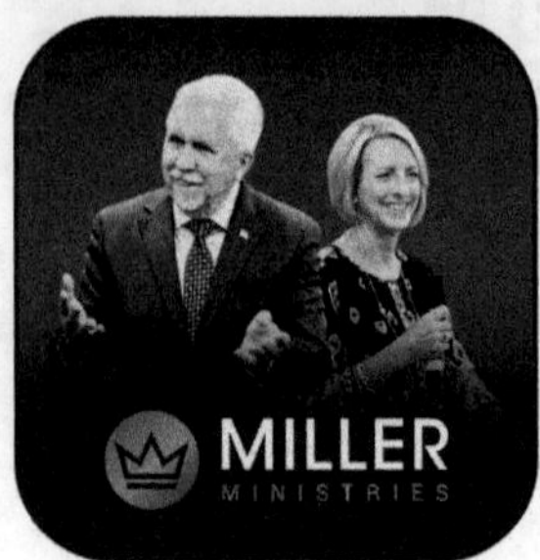

Miller Ministries 

YouTube Channel

Watch faith-building messages from Jeff and Christine Miller, the Miller family, guest ministers, and our livestreamed services. Each video is rooted in God's Word and designed to help you grow in faith, receive healing, and walk in the fullness of His promises.

Christine Miller Podcast 

Available on Apple Podcasts

This audio podcast features powerful teachings to strengthen your faith and help you walk in the victory that belongs to you in Christ. Hear biblical truths such as faith, healing, righteousness, and being led by the Holy Spirit. These clear teachings will renew your mind and build confidence in God's promises.

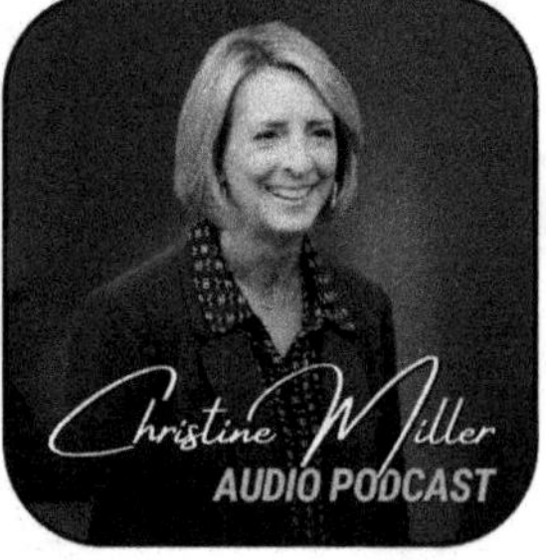

Healing Nuggets 

Weekly Blog Posts

The *Healing Nuggets Blog* provides weekly Scripture-based teaching focused on biblical healing and victorious Christian living. Each blog post is designed to build your faith, renew your mind, and help you receive the healing God has already provided through Christ.

Share Your Testimony 

We'd love to hear what God has been doing in your life! Scan the QR code or visit **millerministries.org/testimony**.

Connect with us! 

youtube.com/millerministries instgram.com/miller_ministries

facebook.com/abundantlifefoxvalley x.com/millermininintl

www.ingramcontent.com/pod-product-compliance
Lightning Source LLC
LaVergne TN
LVHW010704110826
845149LV00014B/3221

* 9 7 8 0 9 8 4 6 9 1 8 7 6 *